Cosmetic and Reconstructive Surgery of Congenital Ear Deformities

Editor

SCOTT STEPHAN

FACIAL PLASTIC SURGERY CLINICS OF NORTH AMERICA

www.facialplastic.theclinics.com

Consulting Editor
J. REGAN THOMAS

February 2018 • Volume 26 • Number 1

ELSEVIER

1600 John F. Kennedy Boulevard • Suite 1800 • Philadelphia, Pennsylvania, 19103-2899

http://www.theclinics.com

FACIAL PLASTIC SURGERY CLINICS OF NORTH AMERICA Volume 26, Number 1
February 2018 ISSN 1064-7406, ISBN-13: 978-0-323-56978-1

Editor: Jessica McCool
Developmental Editor: Meredith Madeira

Facial Plastic Surgery Clinics of North America (ISSN 1064-7406) is published quarterly by Elsevier Inc., 360 Park Avenue South, New York, NY 10010-1710. Months of issue are February, May, August, and November. Business and Editorial Offices: 1600 John F. Kennedy Blvd., Suite 1800, Philadelphia, PA 19103-2899. Periodicals postage paid at New York, NY, and additional mailing offices. Subscription prices are $398.00 per year (US individuals), $628.00 per year (US institutions), $454.00 per year (Canadian individuals), $782.00 per year (Canadian institutions), $535.00 per year (foreign individuals), $782.00 per year (foreign institutions), $100.00 per year (US students), and $255.00 per year (foreign students). Foreign air speed delivery is included in all *Clinics* subscription prices. All prices are subject to change without notice. POSTMASTER: Send address changes to *Facial Plastic Surgery Clinics*, Elsevier Health Sciences Division, Subscription Customer Service, 3251 Riverport Lane, Maryland Heights, MO 63043. **Customer service: 1-800-654-2452 (US and Canada); 1-314-447-8871 (outside US and Canada); Fax: 314-447-8029; E-mail: journalscustomerservice-usa@elsevier.com (for print support); journalsonline support-usa@elsevier.com (for online support).**

Reprints. For copies of 100 or more of articles in this publication, please contact the Commercial Reprints Department, Elsevier Inc., 360 Park Avenue South, New York, NY 10010-1710. Tel.: 212-633-3874; Fax: 212-633-3820; E-mail: reprints@elsevier.com.

Facial Plastic Surgery Clinics of North America is covered in *MEDLINE/PubMed* (*Index Medicus*).

Contributors

CONSULTING EDITOR

J. REGAN THOMAS, MD, FACS
Mansueto Professor and Chairman,
Department of Otolaryngology–Head and Neck
Surgery, University of Illinois at Chicago,
Chicago, Illinois, USA

EDITOR

SCOTT STEPHAN, MD
Assistant Professor, Facial Plastic and
Reconstructive Surgery, Department of
Otolaryngology–Head and Neck Surgery,
Directory of Microtia-Atreisa Clinic, Associate
Fellowship Director, Vanderbilt University
Medical Center, Nashville, Tennessee, USA

AUTHORS

ARTURO BONILLA, MD
Founder and Director, Microtia–Congenital Ear
Deformity Institute, San Antonio, Texas, USA

SIVAKUMAR CHINNADURAI, MD, MPH
Associate Professor, Department of
Otolaryngology, Vanderbilt University Medical
Center, Nashville, Tennessee, USA;
Department of Otolaryngology and Facial
Plastic Surgery, Children's Hospitals and
Clinics of Minnesota, Minneapolis, Minnesota,
USA

PHILIPPE A. FEDERSPIL, MD
Assistant Professor, Department of
Oto-Rhino-Laryngology, Director, Division of
Oncological ENT Surgery, Heidelberg
University Hospital, President, International
Association for Surgical Prosthetics and
Episthetics (IASPE), Heidelberg, Germany

BRADLEY W. KESSER, MD
Professor, Department of
Otolaryngology–Head and Neck Surgery,
University of Virginia School of Medicine,
Charlottesville, Virginia, USA

LUCA LANCEROTTO, MD, PhD
Fellow in Plastic Surgery, Department of
Plastic Surgery, Royal Hospital for Sick
Children, Edinburgh, United Kingdom

CHRISTEN LENNON, MD
Department of Otolaryngology, Vanderbilt
University Medical Center, Nashville,
Tennessee, USA

JIAHUI LIN, MD
Resident, Department of Otolaryngology,
Columbia University Medical Center, Weill
Cornell Medicine, New York, New York, USA

JOHN REINISCH, MD
Professor, Division of Plastic Surgery,
Keck School of Medicine of the University of
Southern California, Los Angeles, California,
California, USA

DOUGLAS S. RUHL, MD, MSPH
Adjunct Assistant Professor, Department
of Otolaryngology–Head and Neck Surgery,
University of Virginia School of Medicine,
Charlottesville, Virginia, USA

ALEXANDER L. SCHNEIDER, MD
Department of Otolaryngology–Head and
Neck Surgery, Northwestern University
Feinberg School of Medicine, Chicago,
Illinois, USA

ANTHONY P. SCLAFANI, MD, FACS
Professor of Otolaryngology, Director of Facial
Plastic Surgery, Weill Cornell Medicine, New
York, New York, USA

DOUGLAS M. SIDLE, MD
Assistant Professor, Department
of Otolaryngology–Head and Neck
Surgery, Northwestern University
Feinberg School of Medicine, Chicago,
Illinois, USA

SCOTT STEPHAN, MD
Assistant Professor, Facial Plastic and
Reconstructive Surgery, Department of
Otolaryngology–Head and Neck Surgery,
Directory of Microtia-Atreisa Clinic, Associate
Fellowship Director, Vanderbilt University
Medical Center, Nashville, Tennessee, USA

**KENNETH J. STEWART, MD,
FRCS(Ed)(Plast)**
Consultant Plastic Surgeon, Department of
Plastic Surgery, Royal Hospital for Sick
Children, Edinburgh, United Kingdom

AKIRA YAMADA, MD, PhD
Professor of Plastic Surgery, World
Craniofacial Foundation, Dallas, Texas, USA

Contents

> Congenital auricular deformities often can be corrected by neonatal ear molding techniques, which have evolved significantly over a 25-year period with commercially available molding systems. Indications for molding and methodology for best optimizing results have been well described in the literature, although recent studies have explored the methodology for reduction in the cost of technique and also called for increased awareness among pediatric practitioners of the importance of early institution of therapy.

> Otoplasty is one of the first procedures learned during residency. A myriad of surgical techniques and nuances exist. Many have merit, some are ineffective, some destructive, and some frankly fanciful. Adopting an effective and safe technique should be based on proven efficacy and effectiveness to avoid early disappointments. The authors present a review of traditional otoplasty techniques and more recent innovations. Their pros and cons are discussed in view of the relative risks/benefits balance. Recurrence rates are low for most techniques. Some techniques carry a higher risk of significant complications. A ladder approach preferring techniques that minimize cartilage damage seems advisable.

> Otoplasty for prominent ears is a rewarding yet exacting surgery that demands the precise application of anatomic knowledge, anthropometric norms, and surgical creativity. The practitioner must be able to use a variety of different techniques to provide durable and acceptable cosmetic results to patients. This article provides an in-depth description of normal and abnormal auricular anatomy and the historical context for modern otoplasty and describes in detail the common otoplastic procedures currently performed.

> Among the less common congenital auricular anomalies are cryptotia, Stahl ear, constricted ear, and macrotia. The vast majority of these occur spontaneously without accompanying syndromes or other deformities. This article provides a comprehensive overview of these anomalies, as well as common techniques to correct these anomalies.

> The Nagata technique is the most popular method of autologous rib microtia construction. To achieve successful outcome, 3 keys must be perfect: the skin envelope, the 3D cartilage framework, and proper location of the construct. The first step of the surgery is to identify the "auricular rectangle." The relationship between the auricular rectangle and the vestige will determine if the vestige is usable for surgery. Rib cartilage must be harvested without perichondrium to prevent chest deformity. Lobule split technique is the hallmark of the Nagata technique, which allows skin envelope expansion, and allows deeper conchal cavity. Surgeons must master the 3D framework construct before clinical cases.

> Reconstruction of the microtic ear is one of the most challenging, yet gratifying, surgical experiences. Careful planning, attention to detail, and conservative tissue management are necessary for excellent results. Technologies continue to evolve; with the advancement of cartilage tissue engineering, the future of ear reconstruction is very promising.

> Alloplast-based ear reconstruction has become more popular over the years because it offers many advantages compared with the traditional staged autologous costal cartilage approach. Advantages include earlier reconstruction in the setting of microtia, fewer procedures, less donor site morbidity, shorter surgeon learning curve, and improved consistency in the final aesthetic result. Although other implantable materials have been used in auricular reconstruction with variable success, porous high-density polyethylene frameworks combined with recent advances in the creation of the soft tissue coverage have significantly improved outcomes with minimal complications and long-term viability. This article describes the authors' technique.

> Patients with microtia and congenital aural atresia should have a comprehensive hearing assessment early in life. Options for hearing habilitation should be presented, and children with bilateral aural atresia should be fitted with a bone conducting hearing device to support normal speech and language development. If atresia surgery is pursued, the microtia surgeon must be aware of certain principles. This article presents recommendations on options for potentially improving hearing in children with congenital aural atresia: assessing surgical candidacy, chronology and timing of surgeries, functional importance of certain ear structures, and understanding the possible locations of an aberrant facial nerve to avoid injury in these patients.

The progress made in the development of the silicones and percutaneous titanium implants allows for rehabilitation of patients with microtia with an inconspicuous auricular prosthesis. The art of making the prosthesis by the dedicated anaplastologist is the key for the success of this approach. Most patients with microtia desire camouflage. The greatest advantage of the auricular prosthesis is that it can be manufactured as a mirrored replica of the opposite side. The outcome is predictable. Computer science with virtual planning and rapid prototyping is about to revolutionize the process of prosthetic auricular rehabilitation.

FACIAL PLASTIC SURGERY CLINICS OF NORTH AMERICA

RELATED INTEREST

Clinics in Sports Medicine, April 2017 (Vol. 36, No. 2)
Facial Injuries in Sports
Michael J. Stuart, *Editor*
Available at: http://www.sportsmed.theclinics.com/

THE CLINICS ARE AVAILABLE ONLINE!
Access your subscription at:
www.theclinics.com

Preface

Cosmetic and Reconstructive Surgery of Congenital Ear Deformities

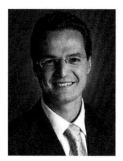

Scott Stephan, MD
Editor

It is my privilege and great pleasure to introduce this issue of *Facial Plastic Surgery Clinics of North America* with a comprehensive focus on cosmetic and reconstructive surgery of congenital ear deformities. First and foremost, I wish to thank sincerely our many wonderful authors who graciously offered their time, commitment, and world-class expertise in this specialty subject for the benefit of our readership.

With its unique blend of individual subtly, three-dimensional detail, and discrete position on the head, surgery to reshape or reconstruct the ear demands a great deal of skill and attention to detail. The complexity of auricular embryology lends itself to the development of a multitude of ear malformations that spans a broad spectrum. Some of these deformities are more pronounced than others, but all are seen through the lens of symmetry with the opposite ear posing a true challenge of comparison to the surgeon.

No matter your age or background, there is no expertise needed to see asymmetry or malformation—it is preprogrammed into human perception to pick out what is different. In the treatment of congenital ear deformities, ultimately our patients want a natural, unremarkable ear that blends the gentle and sudden transitions seen in the exquisite architecture and cast of shadows of a normal ear. It is likely these factors of aesthetic nuance that make reshaping or reconstructing an ear so difficult, and in turn, so rewarding an endeavor for patient and surgeon alike.

There is a detail-oriented discipline needed to diagnose the subtle malformation of an auricular subunit or to recognize the global malposition of a lobule-canal remnant. This calculated methodology then gives way to the creative and often individualized solutions for each patient before finally the technical demands of the surgery are called upon.

Somewhat unique to the ear is the expertise needed to know when to intervene for each kind of problem. Our authors bring attention not just to the technical details of the surgery but also to the considerations that dictate the chronology of care. Furthermore, this issue also reviews how those performing aesthetic ear reconstruction need to consider and accommodate the functional auditory problems that often accompany the

Facial Plast Surg Clin N Am 26 (2018) ix–x
https://doi.org/10.1016/j.fsc.2017.10.001
1064-7406/18/© 2017 Published by Elsevier Inc.

more severe ear malformations. This interphase between aesthetic and functional goals makes the global care of the patient a multidisciplinary endeavor between the aesthetic ear surgeon and other specialties such as audiology, otology, anaplastology, and even maxillofacial surgery. In this way, the treatment of congenital ear malformations has become fertile ground for some of the most exciting areas of innovation in facial plastic surgery.

My hope is that this issue sparks the interest and enjoyment of our readers and conveys the wonderful blend of artistry and ability required for the treatment of congenital ear malformations.

Scott Stephan, MD
Facial Plastic and Reconstructive Surgery
Department of Otolaryngology-Head and
Neck Surgery
Vanderbilt University Medical Center
Nashville, TN 37232, USA

E-mail address:
stephan@vanderbilt.edu

Nonsurgical Management of Congenital Auricular Anomalies

Christen Lennon, MD[a],
Sivakumar Chinnadurai, MD, MPH[a,b],*

KEYWORDS

- Auricular anomalies • Auricular deformities • Auricular malformations • Ear molding

KEY POINTS

- Initiation of ear molding at less than 3 weeks of age is critical to optimize results.
- Various molding strategies are available both commercially and with use of custom molding materials.
- The body of evidence supporting ear molding provides adequate support for routine implementation of this methodology for auricular deformities and select malformations.
- Awareness and early detection are the main barriers to successful treatment of moldable auricular anomalies.

INTRODUCTION

Congenital auricular anomalies are a group of heterogeneous malformations and deformities that are highly variable. Although it has been estimated that 50% of the malformations of the ear, nose, and throat affect the ear,[1] the incidence of congenital auricular anomalies is largely unknown. Reports range from auricular anomalies affecting 1:6000 newborns[2] to 5% of the white population (including prominent ear).[3] Studies usually quote lower rates for malformational auricular anomalies, such as microtia and anotia, with a higher incidence in Hispanic and Asian populations.[4] The discrepancies in incidence are somewhat due to variability based on race; however, these statistics also are dependent on whether less severe ear abnormalities are accounted for.

Auricular deformities are associated with a great deal of psychological morbidity, including distress, anxiety, self-consciousness, behavioral problems, and social avoidance.[5] Encouragingly, studies have demonstrated psychological morbidity associated with anatomic ear deformities improves following surgical correction.[5] Ear molding provides the opportunity to definitively prevent the development of such issues for children born with ear anomalies.

Congenital auricular anomalies may occur either in isolation or as part of a syndrome. Approximately 30% are associated with syndromes involving additional malformations and/or functional loss of organs and organ systems.[1] Examples are otofacial dysostosis (Goldenhar syndrome, Treacher-Collins syndrome), craniofacial dysostosis (Crouzon syndrome, Apert syndrome), otocervical dysostosis, otoskeletal dysostosis, and chromosomal syndromes, such as trisomy 13, trisomy 18, trisomy 21, and 18q syndrome.[1]

Congenital ear anomalies, shown in **Table 1**, are categorized as either malformations (eg, microtia, cryptotia) or deformities (eg, Stahl ear, prominent ear). This classification scheme was proposed by Tan and colleagues[6] in 1997. Ear malformations

Disclosure: C. Lennon and S. Chinnadurai have nothing they wish to disclose.
[a] Department of Otolaryngology, Vanderbilt University Medical Center, 2200 Childrens Way, Nashville, TN 37232, USA; [b] Department of Otolaryngology and Facial Plastic Surgery, Children's Hospitals and Clinic of Minnesota, 2530 Chicago Avenue, Minneapolis, MN 55404, USA
* Corresponding author. Department of Otolaryngology and Facial Plastic Surgery, Children's Hospitals and Clinic of Minnesota, 2530 Chicago Avenue, Minneapolis, MN 55404, USA
E-mail address: siva.chinnadurai@childrensmn.org

Facial Plast Surg Clin N Am 26 (2018) 1–8
https://doi.org/10.1016/j.fsc.2017.09.001

Table 1 Ear lesion classification	
Auricular Deformities	**Auricular Malformations**
Stahl ear	Anotia
Cup ear	Microtia
Lop ear	Cryptotia
Conchal crus	Constricted ear
Helical rim deformity	
Prominent ear	
Ear lidding	

are hypothesized to either be caused by errors in embryologic development between the fifth and the ninth gestational week[7] or by germline mutations.[8] Regardless, these errors cause partial absence of skin and/or cartilage resulting in constricted or underdeveloped pinna and/or supernumerary auricular components. Malformations often require surgical intervention during childhood or adolescence,[9] although in cases of less severe malformation, ear molding can sometimes be applied and be useful.

Ear deformities, on the other hand, are ear anomalies that show an abnormal shape with fully developed chondrocutaneous components. Practically speaking, deformational auricular anomalies are classified as such if the ear can be corrected digitally in to an acceptable shape and position. deformities are thought to result from in utero or ex utero deformational forces, including those caused by an aberrant insertion of the intrinsic or extrinsic auricular muscles.[7] It is these types of anomalies that are best treated with auricular molding.

Children with ear deformities that are not corrected at birth often require surgical correction later in life, typically after 5 or 6 years old, when the auricle is approximately 90% of its adult size. Not only is this delay in treatment frustrating for parents, but it also creates an opportunity for social stigma and poor self-image. Further, otoplasty procedures involve risks such as infection, hematoma, and need for revision surgeries.[10] They are often more costly and associated with worse cosmetic outcome than molding.[10]

There have been efforts toward education of neonatal pediatricians, obstetricians, family medicine doctors, and midwives to better capture patients in need of ear molding, as early management is crucial for optimal results.

HISTORY OF TECHNIQUE

Molding and shaping of tissues has historically been practiced since ancient times. Artificial cranial deformation was practiced commonly by many cultures, where restriction of growth through binding or flattening between 2 pieces of wood was used to create a desirable head shape. This is still practiced today in some places. In Imperial China, foot binding was the custom of applying tight binding to the feet of young girls to modify the shape of the foot. Feet altered by binding were called lotus feet, and were a means of displaying social status in ancient Chinese culture.

The use of molding force has been applied in modern medicine in such areas as conventional orthodontics, treatment of congenital hip dislocation, and with the Ponseti casting method for congenital clubfoot correction. More recently, the institution of nasoalveolar molding has decreased the severity of malformation and optimized cleft surgery outcomes.

Using the principle of use of molding force, namely that antagonistic forces create auricular deformities, and also taking advantage of neonatal cartilage's high plasticity, various nonsurgical corrections using opposing forces to reverse or reduce auricular deformities in the early newborn period have been described. Plastic surgeons in Japan first published reports of nonsurgical correction of congenital auricular deformities in 1984.[11,12] This was achieved using splinting the ear with foam. Studies have since described molding using a variety of techniques, using flexible silicone tubing covering stainless steel wire,[9] Reston foam, dental compounds, and coated electrical wire (see Application of Custom or Prefabricated Wire section for more information on the use of these materials). Commercially available prefabricated molding devices have also been developed including the EarWell Infant Ear Correction System (Becon Medical Ltd, Naperville, IL) and EarBuddies.

Finally, the principle of biological creep is a core plastic surgery principle, describing a phenomenon whereby a stretching force chronically placed on tissue causes stretch-induced signal transduction pathways to trigger an increased production of collagen, epidermal proliferation, fibroblast mitosis, and angiogenesis. This principle is historically applied in conventional tissue expansion; however, some authors describe ear molding of constricted and cryptotia ear malformations using this principle as well. This article was the first to describe molding of malformed ears using the classification described by Tan and colleagues[6] in 1997.

CURRENT METHODOLOGY
Timing of Molding

Although various commercial and office-made devices are presently used to correct neonatal ear anomalies, it is widely agreed that time of treatment initiation is the single most important factor in success.[13] High levels of maternal estrogen are present in fetal blood immediately after birth and are hypothesized to influence the malleability of the auricular cartilage in the early newborn period. These levels typically peak within 72 hours after birth and decline steadily over the coming weeks. Hyaluronic acid, which is an important component of ear cartilage, is increased by estrogen and increases its plasticity. As the circulating levels of estrogen decrease in the weeks after birth, the auricle becomes more elastic and firm.[14]

Molding has been shown to be most effective when splinting is started within the first 3 weeks of life. When starting within this window, success rates as determined by parental report are as high as 93%. Outcomes are less favorable if treatment is initiated after 3 weeks.[10,13] Further, it has been suggested by Doft and colleagues[10] that if molding is initiated in the first week of life, the total treatment time can be shortened substantially.

Historically, ear molding has been applied outside of the neonatal period, and the literature has several case series of molding older children, even into teenage years. In general, these investigators used rigid fixation or traction, required long courses of molding, and had markedly less favorable results with a higher incidence of local wound complications.[6,15–17] Currently, delayed molding is not a common practice, with Daniali and colleagues[18] citing a 50% failure rate for molding initiated after 3 weeks of age.

Patient Selection

Aside from timing, the type of ear anomaly is a significant factor in patient selection. Early studies of ear molding efficacy were limited to children with ear deformities only (see **Table 1** for a description of auricular deformities and malformations). As previously noted, recent literature supports the expansion of patient selection to include those with mild ear malformations.[18] Molding still yields unsatisfactory results in more than mild malformations.

Available Molds

A variety of materials have been successfully customized to mold infants' ears. Most commonly, the custom-made splints of metal wire (20–24-gauge dental wire) in silastic tubing, thermoplastic dental impression material, tape, and small bolsters. Examples of custom molding materials are shown in **Fig. 1**. These devices are affixed to the ear with cyanoacetate glue or tape. The use of custom-made molds is attractive because the materials are familiar, easily available, and very inexpensive. They also may be better able to address conchal bowl and inferior rim/lobular anomalies. The notable shortcoming of most custom-made molds is that all molding takes place on the lateral surface of the ear. This is useful for anomalies of the helical rim, conchal crus, and prominent ear. It is not as useful for deepening of the scapha, creation of a well-defined and projected superior crus, or a well-defined triangular fossa.

More recently, prefabricated molding systems (eg, EarWell [Beacon Medical, Naperville, IL] and EarBuddies [Earbuddies, London, England]) have become widely available and offer the convenience of a variety of molding tools without the time-consuming process of creating custom devices for each application. Although some are more polished versions of wire-based molding, others allow for customizable 3-dimensional molding offering

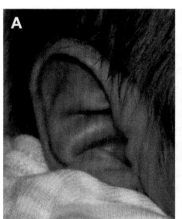 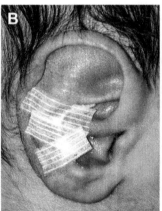 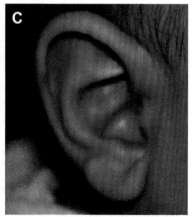

Fig. 1. Custom splinting photos. Custom splint using dental wire and silastic tubing for treatment of prominent conchal crus. (*A*) Before molding. (*B*) With custom molding materials in place. (*C*) After removal of custom molding materials.

the advantage of molding the ear both laterally and medially, which allows more control over deepening the scapha and the creation of a defined superior crus. Fixation is also more rigid, which allows the ability to treat more complex ear lesions, including mild malformations (**Fig. 2**).

Technique

Informed consent is obtained from parents, specifically citing the possibility of skin breakdown, local wound infection, failure to achieve the desired cosmetic result, and the need for further procedures (see the Complications section for further details on this topic).

Children within the first 2 to 3 weeks of life will often sleep through the procedure, and a simple swaddle is usually sufficient for immobilization. In older infants, a papoose board is used as needed. It is often helpful to advise families to feed their infants shortly before the procedure and have a pacifier ready if the child uses one. An assistant sits across the table to help with positioning of the child's head. If any portion of the molding application is to contact hair-bearing skin, the area of anticipated adhesion is meticulously shaved. Any hair in the distribution of the adhesive will both make the molding device less stable and more likely to prematurely detach.

Application of EarWell Prefabricated Molding Device

The senior author (SC) most commonly uses prefabricated molding devices, which are applicable to a wide range of ear anomalies. Following hair removal, the mold is "dry fitted" to see how it best sits with relation to the ear and internal retractors are bent to the appropriate shape. The skin is then cleaned with 2 applications of rubbing alcohol. Each is allowed 30 seconds to dry. This time is used to remove the paper tabs over the adhesive to break the strong bond that is present out of the packaging. The paper tabs are then loosely replaced so that they are easier to remove when the device is in place.

After the alcohol has dried, the external cradle is placed with the tape still in place. It is adjusted until it is sitting in the desired position, then the tape is removed. Once attached to the skin, gentle pressure is held around the circumference of the device for several seconds to ensure complete adhesion to the skin. Previously shaped internal retractors are applied and a cap is placed over the cradle.

Application of Custom or Prefabricated Wire

The authors use custom-made splints from 8-Fr suction tubing and 22 to 24-gauge dental wire in instances in which the lesion may be difficult to control with prefabricated devices. These include far anterior helical root constriction or lidding, or very prominent conchal crus.

Before preparing the skin, an appropriately sized splint is created. Wire is cut to length and inserted into the silicone tubing, which is then cut 1 mm longer so the wire does not protrude from the end. The ends of the tubing are sealed with a piece of tape and the device is then bent into the desired shape. Skin preparation then proceeds as detailed in the previous section, including skin preparation with alcohol and hair removal if needed.

After the alcohol has dried, a very thin layer of liquid adhesive (Mastisol; Eloquest Healthcare, Ferndale, MI) is applied over the area where the wire will be and where tape will contact the skin. When this has dried, the wire is applied and the shape and position are verified. The wire is then secured with several one-quarter-inch adhesive strips. The use of several small strips allows tension in several directions.

Treatment Course

When started in the ideal time window of younger than 3 weeks of age, a typical course of molding is 6 weeks. Typically, children are followed at 2-week intervals with assessment for skin complications and replacement of the molding device at each visit. In children with more complex lesions, such as cryptotia, the goal of the first splint application is retraction of the cartilage out from under the temporoparietal skin with planned shaping of the auricle in later applications. In these situations, more frequent follow-up may be indicated.

Complications

Byrd and colleagues[13] described minor complications in 5% of the infants treated with EarWell. These included localized skin excoriations or breakdown without cartilage erosion, which were caused by the posterior cradle of the EarWell system becoming loose and reportedly allowing the movement and malposition of the internal parts of the system. In their 2017 study, this group recommended temporary suspension of the helical rim retractor expansion for 5 to 7 days in the face of such excoriations. Another complication described was a monilia skin infection in the area under the adhesive from the EarWell device.

EVIDENCE

Overall, the body of literature concerning the molding of congenital ear deformities is somewhat

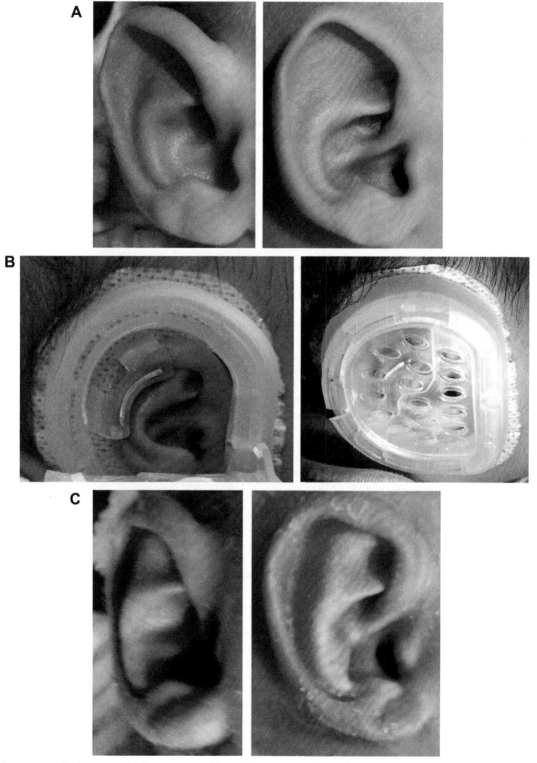

Fig. 2. EarWell photos. EarWell treatment of broad flattened scaphae, absent superior crus, and poorly defined fossa triangularis. (*A*) Before molding. (*B*) With EarWell system in place. (*C*) After removal of EarWell device.

weak in its level of evidence. Most studies concerning ear molding offer descriptive evidence and are presented as case series. There are, however, a few large series published that are described here.

In 2010, Byrd and colleagues[13] published a review of their experience in managing more than 831 ear deformities in 488 patients. They described the evolution of their approach to the timing of ear molding, ultimately adopting a methodology of initial observation for infants seen at birth with reevaluation at 5 to 7 days. This group adopted this approach after observing that approximately one-third of infants with ear deformities showed tendency toward self-correction. Most deformed ears that were evaluated had prominent/cup ear and lidding/lop ear. Most patients presented with bilateral deformities (70%). Finally, this study was the first description of the EarWell system, and Byrd and colleagues[13] reported a success rate of more than 90% (n = 58).

In 2017, this same group published their experience in treating both ear deformities and malformations from 2011 to 2014 with the EarWell system.[18] A total of 303 newborn ear deformities and 175 malformations were treated. The mean age for initiation of ear molding was 12.5 days, with an average adjusted gestational age at initiation of treatment of 39.2 weeks. Duration of treatment ranged from 12 to 109 days, with the average being 37 days. "Retention taping" (affixing a retractor to the helical rim in the area of prior deformity and attaching it to a double-sided tape affixed to the retroauricular skin) was used in 66% of patients for a mean of 1.8 weeks.

In this study, a wide range of deformities was treated: conchal crus (26.4%), helical rim abnormalities (24.8%), (20.8%), lidding (19.0%), and prominent ear (9.0%). Approximately one-third of ears presented with more than one identifiable deformity. Daniali and colleagues[18] reported very good outcomes overall, with 95.1% of conchal crus deformities, 97.5% of helical rim deformities, 97.0% of Stahl's ears, 93.2% of lidded ears, and 88.0% of prominent ears graded as having attained an excellent to good outcome after molding with the EarWell system. Of all the deformities treated, the prominent ear had the greatest number of ears with retained residual deformity (19.6%).

In Daniali's study, 98% of ear malformations were constricted ear, with the remainder of the ears having cryptotia. Cup ear was considered a variant of the constricted ear. Constriction was significantly improved, as evidenced by a reduction in constriction severity class by, on average, 1.24 points (P<.01). Overall posttreatment outcomes were graded as excellent to good in 88.2% of constricted ears as reported by surgeon opinion of blinded photographs. Importantly, patients with malformations were seen weekly rather than biweekly to advance the treatment, but also to monitor for abrasion or irritation from the increased pressure and tension being applied. Complication rate in the deformational group was similar to that experienced in the malformational group (7.2% vs 8.1%, respectively).

Doft and colleagues[10] published a prospective study on 158 ears that underwent molding with the EarWell system. Eighty-two percent of the children had the device placed in the newborn nursery and 95% had it placed before 2 weeks of life. Average treatment time was 14 days, and 96% of the deformities were corrected; however, the time point of this observation is unclear. Parents were surveyed following treatment, and 99% stated that they would have the procedure repeated. The importance of early initiation (most within the first week of life) of therapy was highlighted in this study, with their average treatment time significantly lower than what had previously been described in the literature.

The most recent robust literature review was published in 2009 by van Wijk and colleagues.[19]

Twenty studies were included from a literature search performed in July 2008. This article called attention to the fact that much is still unknown regarding indications for splinting, as it is largely unknown what proportion of ear deformities resolve spontaneously after birth. One early study by Matsuo and colleagues[11] did show that.

Further review of the literature reveals smaller studies supporting the overall findings of those described previously.[6,9,20–22] Three studies by Tan and colleagues[6,12,15] describe molding in older children; however, their results showed substantially poorer outcomes with increased age.

CHALLENGES AND CONTROVERSIES

Knowledge about timing of mold application continues to evolve. Although it is generally well agreed on that younger infants have better results and shorter treatment courses than older infants, debate still exists about whether to splint children in the first week of life. The proportion of anomalies that self-resolve is unknown, raising concern of overtreatment for mild anomalies.

As early identification is the major barrier to treating children with these lesions, there also is not a firm consensus on when it is too late for molding. Current practice offers estimates ranging from 4 weeks to 3 months as the latest date that neonatal molding can successfully be applied.

Finally, the current base of literature relies almost entirely on subjective reporting. There is no standard or validated tool to assess neonatal ear anomalies, and practitioners often evaluate their own results or rely on parent self-report or evaluation by their colleagues. This approach offers some internal validity, but there is little external validity to compare different techniques and molding lengths across studies, limiting the strength of evidence around this topic.

FUTURE DIRECTIONS

The most critical issue in the future of ear molding is raising awareness of treatable ear anomalies and the time frame in which they should be treated. In the authors' institution, this is achieved by twice-yearly teaching sessions with newborn hearing screeners. In this way, many molding candidates are identified within the first 3 days of life and offered a clinic referral or inpatient consult. The approach to this at individual institutions may differ.

Select investigators have called for attention to be drawn to congenital auricular anomalies as a public health issue rather than a surgical problem. Although this argument underscores the need for early identification of easily correctable deformities, this statement has been used to justify an argument for primary care practitioners to initiate molding therapy themselves with a referral to specialists for support if necessary. It is our opinion that although primary care physicians can be instrumental in early identification, ear molding is a distinct skillset that is not easily acquired unless practiced in a large volume. For these reasons, we would advocate for early referral to a specialist for optimal care of these children.

The body of evidence around ear molding would benefit from further assessment of the cutoff point for neonatal ear molding and more homogeneity in judging outcomes to allow for comparison across studies and techniques. Furthermore, it may be beneficial for future studies regarding ear molding to include more long-term follow-up to investigate outcomes as they relate to need for further surgical intervention later in life.

REFERENCES

1. Bartel-Friedrich S, Wulke C. Classification and diagnosis of ear malformations. GMS Curr Top Otorhinolaryngol Head Neck Surg 2007;6:Doc05.
2. Brent B. The pediatrician's role in caring for patients with congenital microtia and atresia. Pediatr Ann 1999;28(6):374–83.
3. Songu M, Kutlu A. Long-term psychosocial impact of otoplasty performed on children with prominent ears. J Laryngol Otol 2014;128(9):768–71.
4. Harris J, Kallen B, Robert E. The epidemiology of anotia and microtia. J Med Genet 1996;33(10):809–13.
5. Horlock N, Vogelin E, Bradbury ET, et al. Psychosocial outcome of patients after ear reconstruction: a retrospective study of 62 patients. Ann Plast Surg 2005;54(5):517–24.
6. Tan ST, Abramson DL, MacDonald DM, et al. Molding therapy for infants with deformational auricular anomalies. Ann Plast Surg 1997;38(3):263–8.
7. Porter CJ, Tan ST. Congenital auricular anomalies: topographic anatomy, embryology, classification, and treatment strategies. Plast Reconstr Surg 2005;115(6):1701–12.
8. Artunduaga MA, Quintanilla-Dieck Mde L, Greenway S, et al. A classic twin study of external ear malformations, including microtia. N Engl J Med 2009;361(12):1216–8.
9. Mohammadi AA, Imani MT, Kardeh S, et al. Non-surgical management of congenital auricular deformities. World J Plast Surg 2016;5(2):139–47.
10. Doft MA, Goodkind AB, Diamond S, et al. The newborn butterfly project: a shortened treatment protocol for ear molding. Plast Reconstr Surg 2015;135(3):577e–83e.
11. Matsuo K, Hirose T, Tomono T, et al. Nonsurgical correction of congenital auricular deformities in the early neonate: a preliminary report. Plast Reconstr Surg 1984;73(1):38–51.
12. Tan ST, Shibu M, Gault DT. A splint for correction of congenital ear deformities. Br J Plast Surg 1994;47(8):575–8.
13. Byrd HS, Langevin CJ, Ghidoni LA. Ear molding in newborn infants with auricular deformities. Plast Reconstr Surg 2010;126(4):1191–200.
14. Anstadt EE, Johns DN, Kwok AC, et al. Neonatal ear molding: timing and technique. Pediatrics 2016;137(3):e20152831.
15. Tan S, Wright A, Hemphill A, et al. Correction of deformational auricular anomalies by moulding–results of a fast-track service. N Z Med J 2003;116(1181):U584.
16. Yotsuyanagi T, Yokoi K, Sawada Y. Nonsurgical treatment of various auricular deformities. Clin Plast Surg 2002;29(2):327–32, ix.
17. Yotsuyanagi T. Nonsurgical correction of congenital auricular deformities in children older than early neonates. Plast Reconstr Surg 2004;114(1):190–1.
18. Daniali LN, Rezzadeh K, Shell C, et al. Classification of newborn ear malformations and their treatment with the earwell infant ear correction system. Plast Reconstr Surg 2017;139(3):681–91.

19. van Wijk MP, Breugem CC, Kon M. Non-surgical correction of congenital deformities of the auricle: a systematic review of the literature. J Plast Reconstr Aesthet Surg 2009;62(6):727–36.

20. Chang CS, Bartlett SP. A simplified nonsurgical method for the correction of neonatal deformational auricular anomalies. Clin Pediatr (Phila) 2017;56(2): 132–9.

21. Ullmann Y, Blazer S, Ramon Y, et al. Early nonsurgical correction of congenital auricular deformities. Plast Reconstr Surg 2002;109(3):907–13 [discussion: 914–5].

22. Woo T, Kim YS, Roh TS, et al. Correction of congenital auricular deformities using the ear-molding technique. Arch Plast Surg 2016;43(6): 512–7.

Surgical Otoplasty
An Evidence-Based Approach to Prominent Ears Correction

Kenneth J. Stewart, MD, FRCS(Ed)(Plast)*,
Luca Lancerotto, MD, PhD

KEYWORDS

- Otoplasty • Prominent ear • Evidence • Posterior suturing • Anterior scoring • Suture
- Complications • Incisionless

KEY POINTS

- Prominent ear correction techniques can be distinguished in cartilage-sculpting (incision or scoring) versus cartilage-sparing (suture techniques).
- Cartilage-sculpting techniques can occasionally result in sharp edges and difficult-to-treat deformities.
- Posterior suturing recurrence and suture-related complications are minimized by the adoption of a fascial flap technique with vest-over-pants wound closure.
- Posterior suturing has lower risks of noncorrectible cartilage distortion or disruption.

INTRODUCTION

In the Western world, requests for interventions to improve the appearance of the ears are common. Otoplasty accounted for 1.3% of plastic surgical interventions performed in 2016 by US plastic surgeons,[1] 3.2% in the United Kingdom,[2] and 2.6% worldwide in 2015.[3] These statistics do not consider procedures performed by specialists other than plastic surgeons. In general, these procedures present low risk with favorable patient outcomes. However, significant complications and litigations can and do occur.

For many plastic surgeons, otoplasty techniques are often learned early in training. A myriad of techniques and nuances of surgical techniques exist in the literature. Many have merit, some are ineffective, some are destructive, and some are frankly fanciful. For the resident in training and the newly established independent practitioner, adopting an effective and safe technique should not merely be secondary to the influence of her or his trainers but should be based on proven efficacy and effectiveness to avoid early disappointments. Above all, beware the latest fad or the latest marketing campaign.

PATIENT ASSESSMENT

Patients present across the entire age range requesting correction of prominent ears. Some degree of ear deformity is common at birth, affecting 55.2% of newborns in a Japanese study examining 1000 infants.[4] However, only 0.4% of ears are regarded as prominent at birth. A Canadian study on 800 newborns identified a much smaller incidence of general deformity (6%), but a similar 0.75% incidence of ear protrusion.[5] Although ear deformities largely self-resolve, ear prominence increases to 5.5% at 1 year.[4] Parents, often driven

Disclosure Statement: K.J. Stewart and L. Lancerotto have nothing they wish to disclose.
Department of Plastic Surgery, Royal Hospital for Sick Children, 9 Sciennes Road, Edinburgh EH9 1LF, UK
* Corresponding author.
E-mail address: ken.stewart2@nhs.net

Facial Plast Surg Clin N Am 26 (2018) 9–18
https://doi.org/10.1016/j.fsc.2017.09.002

by Internet searches or on recommendation of professionals, will present with enquiries about ear splinting.[6–8]

The ethics of operating on children are complex. Parents will frequently request intervention before school to "prevent teasing and bullying," yet we have no evidence that early intervention provides any protection against the psychological rigors of childhood. Others will argue that children should have reached an age of competence so that they can be an arbiter of their own ear fate. To operate on all children who present with prominent ears is, without doubt, to operate on many unnecessarily. For some, prominent ears will eventually become problematic enough to warrant intervention. Others will cope perfectly and will not be affected in their social, educational, or occupational inter- actions. A review of successful individuals in pub- lic life quickly negates the notion that prominent ears are a barrier to success.

Some have extrapolated the cleft palate debate to otoplasty. Early intervention in cleft palate is necessary, but is clearly associated with poorer midfacial growth. And, thus, early intervention before ear growth may adversely affect growth. However, evidence suggests early otoplasty does not significantly interfere with ear growth. Balogh and Millesi[9] reported on 76 patients having undergone antihelical fold correction by cartilage excision and suturing at the age of 5 to 8 years and reexamined them at 20 to 30 years old. No evident deficiency in ear growth out of normal ranges was noticed when compared against stan- dard measures and against a control cohort. Gosain and colleagues[10] described a case series of 12 patients undergoing otoplasty by cartilage incision and suturing before age 3 and similarly found no effect on ear development at follow-up ranging from 21 months to 7.5 years.

However, a lack of effect on growth does not justify the practice of early otoplasty. Our personal experience suggests a higher incidence of postop- erative difficulties in young children, and a higher adverse psychological burden related to the trau- matic event is a possibility.

We have tried, and probably failed, to add some sense to the difficult question of the "ideal age" for ear surgery.[11] In truth, long-term outcome studies do not exist to substantiate a preferential benefit of surgery at any particular age. Current work to develop standardized ear-related patient-reported outcome measures, such as the EAR-Q, will at least give us the tools to develop such studies.[12,13]

In adults, in theory, no such anxieties exist regarding competence in decision making, yet pitfalls abound. We have all met patients who have exploited the wonders of double-sided sticky tape or superglue to self-correct. Such self-prescribed interventions may not necessarily indicate body dysmorphic disorder (BMD) in as much that the well-groomed young man with bleached teeth, bronzed skin, and ripped muscles necessarily harbors such a diagnosis. Yet studies suggest that the incidence of BMD in facial plastic surgery cases is relatively high. Certainly young surgeons should avoid the temptation to be flat- tered by patients who have traveled a long way to get to their office. Surgical itinerants wearing hats to hide their ears, who disparage every other surgeon they have met, rarely make good surgical candidates.

ANATOMY

A careful evaluation of the anatomy of each ear is essential. Excessive ear projection is the most common complaint. A nonmargined ruler is used to measure the distance between the mastoid and the most prominent point of the helix. Typical findings in aesthetically attractive ears are be- tween 17 and 23 mm. Beyond 25 mm, ears are more frequently regarded as prominent.

Evaluation of ear length and symmetry is neces- sary. In our ear reconstruction practice, we regard the normal range as between 50 mm and 70 mm in length. Numbers are not all. An appreciation of how the ear fits to the face is critical: greater ear length may more readily complement a longer face. Individual components of ear length are also relevant. Excess ear lobule size or length in particular should be noted. Finally, the normal ten- dency for ears to elongate in later life should be appreciated.[14] Older patients may request ear reduction as a rejuvenation procedure.

The anatomic anomalies contributing toward ear prominence should be assessed. The most frequent finding is a relatively obtuse antihelix and superior crus. The inferior crus is less frequently implicated but should be evaluated. In the past, a "deep" conchal bowl was implicated as a common culprit for ear prominence, and conchal reduction surgery was frequently prac- ticed. We now believe this represents an overdiag- nosis of conchal bowl excess. We and others have observed that in the vast majority of cases the conchal bowl is normal in size but is rather rotated in an anterior direction.

Our understanding of the contribution of the various extrinsic and intrinsic ear musculature to ear prominence is in its infancy. A significant pro- portion of patients with acquired facial palsy develop acquired ear prominence, and it will be interesting to elucidate the role of auricular muscu- lature in the development of prominent ears.

Ethnic differences in ear anatomy exist but more significant are the differing aesthetic ideals to which different cultures aspire. In Southeast Asia, for example, perhaps under the influence of Buddhism, prominent ears and large lobules are regarded as lucky and associated with wealth and happiness.

PROMINENT EAR CORRECTION TECHNIQUES

Ear correction techniques are broadly divided between cartilage-sculpting and cartilage-sparing. Some techniques rely on a combination of the 2. More specifically, we identify cutting, scoring, and suturing techniques. This is clearly an over-simplification. Almost every surgeon will have developed his or her preferred technique combining different approaches, which makes it difficult to compare available studies. In addition, nonsurgical techniques are available (splinting), and new options are emerging.

Cartilage-Cutting Techniques

Cutting techniques recreate the prominence of the antihelix by a combination of cartilage incision, excision, and mobilization through a posterior access that builds on the method proposed by Luckett in 1910.[9,15] An even simpler and older way of reducing ear protrusion is the excision of a wedge of cartilage from the concha. This was commonly performed with an anterior approach, in which a less generous wedge of skin was also excised along with cartilage. Modern investigators have occasionally revived such methods.[16–18]

Converse and colleagues[19,20] introduced the concept of cartilage tubing to recreate missing folds. They produced antihelical and superior crus tubing by means of parallel nonjoining full-thickness incisions of the cartilage along the outlines of desired folds via a posterior access. Folding was maintained by sutures and by relying on the splinting effect of postauricular skin excision. In reviewing 570 operated ears over 20 years, Baker and Converse[21] observed a 0.8% incidence of hematoma, 1.2% infections, 2.6% recurrence, 3% telephone deformity, and an unreported number of helix disappearance behind the antihelix.

Too often incisions of the cartilage lead to an unnaturally sharp profile of the new prominences, including the Converse tubing technique, which attracted widespread criticism to these methods. All of these techniques significantly weaken the cartilage frame and potentially lead to deformities that may be difficult to correct.

It is advisable that anterior incisions are limited as much as possible and cartilage excision be performed only in cases of macrotia. When conchal overprojection requires reduction, a posterior approach seems preferable, and excess anterior skin slowly reabsorbs.

Anterior Scoring or Burring

The description by Gibson and Davis[22] of interlocking intracartilaginous forces led to the development of techniques aimed at weakening the anterior cartilaginous surface to allow accentuation of the antihelix. This technique is generally ascribed to Stenstroem[23] and Chongchet.[24] In theory, this may provide a more permanent correction of the prominence; however, the technique principally addresses the antihelix and unless hybridized with another method is poorly predictable with a tendency to overcorrect the antihelix while neglecting the conchal contribution.

Most commonly, a posterior approach is used. Stenstroem's[23] technique accesses the anterior surface by dividing the cauda helicis from the concha. Most investigators now expose the anterior surface by an incision through the scapha at the junction to the helix, thus disconnecting the helical rim from the scapha. This disrupts biomechanical stability and may cause secondary deformities such as the hidden helix, a kinked helical rim, and a long, narrow ear.

Alternatively, an anterior approach through a small skin incision hidden in the helical rim can be used.[25] A tunnel is created in the subperichondral plane, and the anterior cartilaginous surface is scored along the curved lines of desired folding. Alternative methods of anterior weakening have been described. These include needle scoring,[26,27] rasp,[25] scalpel,[24] diamond-coated files,[25] and the use of a guarded burr. Throughout the process of scoring, the cartilage frame should remain intact to avoid sharp ridges. Incisions that are too deep can result in overcorrection.[23] If the cartilage is inadvertently incised full thickness, this should be repaired with stitches.[27] Some techniques, such as rasping, have higher risk of incising through the cartilage or producing irregularities of the anterior surface.[25]

Stenstroem[23] excised a skin ellipse from the postauricular surface and relied on its splinting effect to maintain the tubing of the weakened antihelix, essentially stabilized by scarring. Interestingly, notwithstanding the principle on which the technique is based, he did not expect to observe immediate cartilage folding after scoring, and when he omitted skin excision, a high recurrence rate was observed.[23] Raunig[25] does not excise postauricular skin, but tapes the ear to the mastoid skin for 6 weeks. Thus, it appears that the fibrocartilaginous scarring that remodels the scored surface[28] is the main factor in stabilizing antihelix tubing. In reviewing 302 anterior scoring otoplasties, Raunig[25] identified 3 recurrences, although in 23 ears posterior suturing was combined with the primary procedure and a conchal strip was resected in 4 cases.[25]

A further disadvantage is the necessity to deglove the anterior skin. This increases the risk of hematoma and anterior skin necrosis with delayed healing. The skin in the upper third of the antihelix is particularly thin, and the extensive undermining in this area decreases blood supply.[29] Particular care is required to avoid any undue pressure from dressings.

Chongchet[24] performed a more invasive access by degloving the entire anterior surface of the antehelix and crura, through a posterior skin incision and with a cartilage incision running along almost the entire length of the helical rim. There is a definite risk of helix deformation. Calder and Naasan[30] guard against prolonging the incision anteriorly to the scapha. Prolonging it through the helix in an attempt to overcome spring resistance[31] can result in "Spock"-type ear deformity. Scoring is performed by partially incising the anterior surface with a knife along the lines of the desired folds. In 1039 ears in 562 patients, Calder and Nasaan[30] reported 2.0% hemorrhage, 5.2% infection, 2.1% pathologic scarring, 1.4% skin necrosis, and 8.0% residual deformity. Overall complication rates, and residual deformity in particular, was halved if the operation had been performed by a consultant rather than a resident.[30] Caouette-Laberge and colleagues[29] reported on 500 consecutive cases of anterior scoring performed with the technique described by Crikelair and Cosman.[32] This is a modification of Chongchet's,[24] in which scoring is performed along multiple crossing directions. Of approximately one-third of patients who presented at follow-up, 4.4% had residual deformity. At long-term review, patients reported a 4.4% incidence of abnormal ear shape and 18.3% asymmetry, much higher than observed at postoperative follow-up. As no sutures are used, this might be a sign of progressive recurrence over time. Furthermore, 5.7% of patients had persisting pain, and an additional 7.5% hypersensitivity to cold or touch, whereas 3.9% experienced hyposensitivity at 2 years from surgery. This mirrors the results of the original authors on 89 ears, with 18.0% fair and 15.7% poor outcomes.

Interestingly, many investigators who describe anterior scoring actually hybridize it with posterior suturing.[33–37] Bulstrode and colleagues[27] reviewed the results in 214 ears in 144 patients treated by percutaneous anterior scoring with a bent needle and posterior suturing with skin excision. Complications included 1 case of bleeding, 4 early signs of infection, and 2 hypertrophic scars, all settled uneventfully; 5.3% of patients complained of residual deformity due to undercorrection of the upper pole, whereas 1 patient (0.9%) developed recurrence. The incidence of other complications seems in line with that reported for other techniques and summarized by Calder and Naasan.[30]

Indeed, a combination of both cartilage weakening and posterior suturing can be expected to guarantee the lowest rate of recurrence and increased reliability, as any cartilaginous force against the sutures is removed. However, it also carries the combined risks of the 2 methods.

Posterior Suturing

Popularization of this technique is variously ascribed to Mustardé[38,39] or Furnas,[40] depending on residence west or east of the Atlantic. Mustardé[38,39] described posterior suturing to fold the antihelix, as an evolution of Converse's technique in which no cartilage incisions are performed. Furnas[40] proposed adding conchomastoid sutures. In any event, the basics of the technique have been around for many years with varying degrees of popularity.

Although the precise details vary, the basic principle of most suturing techniques is an incision on the posterior aspect of the ear and the insertion of nonabsorbable sutures to address the relative obtuse antihelical rim and upper crus, as well as the anterior rotation of the conchal bowl. Most commonly, 2 separate rows to sutures are inserted to address these issues individually. At the inferior extent of the antihelix, a further suture may be inserted across the incisura to bring the lobule into alignment. Excision of a postauricular skin ellipse has long been given a prominent role for a supposed splinting effect while scarring occurs. Some authors prefer a dumbbell-shaped excision to prevent telephone deformity. More recent experience indicates no advantage with skin excision.[41] Excess skin redrapes quickly. Furthermore, skin excision carries some risk of overresection, which increases skin suture tension and the likelihood of wound-healing complications and in the worst-case scenario results in difficult-to-revise overcorrection.

Most investigators fold the antihelix with 3 to 4 horizontal mattress sutures and use 2 to 3 conchomastoid sutures. Excessively wide mattress sutures result in undesired transverse pull that deforms the cartilage, especially if pliable. Some prefer much smaller bites and an increased number of sutures.[42]

Sutures have a maximum effect if correctly positioned at the inflection lines of the cartilage. If the 2 antihelical bites are too close together, folding will require a much stronger pull against cartilage resistance, increasing the chances of cheesewiring and recurrence. The most cranial part of the auricle must be corrected by a high suture folding the superior crus in a transverse manner. In some instances, a further suture can be positioned between the triangular fossa and the mastoid fascia. A second row of sutures between the conchal bowl and premastoid fascia affords desirable rotation of the concha. Optimal placement on the conchal lateral wall is required. Rarely in very prominent or stiff conchal bows, anterior rotation alone is insufficient, and excision of a cartilage crescent from the lateral wall is required.

Posterior suturing techniques have the advantage in that degloving of the anterior skin and exposure of the anterior cartilage is not required. Thus, the risk of anterior skin necrosis or anterior hematoma is negated. The disadvantage is the reliance on sutures to hold the ear. Absorbable sutures such as PDS are probably associated with a higher recurrence rate,[43] whereas monofilament nonabsorbables (clear prolene or nylon) have a higher knot-related extrusion rate (reviewed in Limandjaja and colleagues[44]), tend to slip if the knot is close-cut, and are more likely to cheesewire through the cartilage. A round-bodied needle minimizes "cheesewiring" of the cartilage. Full-thickness cartilage bites incorporating the anterior perichondrium also reduce the chances of cheesewiring. Furnas sutures need to be passed deeply through the mastoid fascia, otherwise conchal prominence is likely to recur. Correct positioning is confirmed by strong resistance when pulled.

Sutures too superficial in the skin might extrude and become infected. Some investigators advocate a percutaneous suturing technique to increase control on positioning the suture above the perichondrium.[37] We find that with posterior suturing, adequate infiltration of the anterior surface with local anesthetics and adrenaline results in hydrodissection of the subcutaneous space, which allows for easier transcartilaginous suturing while preventing skin transfixation. Silk sutures, as described by Mustardé, are associated with high complication rates.[45] In Rigg's[46] series, a polyester suture was associated with 7.9% granuloma incidence, all at the antihelical fold. Other investigators report extrusion rates in the same range. Polyester suture can take 12 to 24 months to extrude, and suture removal at that stage does not lead to recurrence.[47]

Suture extrusion may be minimized by raising a medially based flap of superficial muscular aponeurotic system fascia to facilitate a double-breasted closure.[48,49] Basat and colleagues[50] propose a laterally based dermal flap to be anchored to the mastoid periosteum. Since we adopted Horlock and Gault's double-breasted flaps,[48] our rate of suture-related complications has dropped,[41] and we have now settled on the use of braided nonabsorbable 4 to 0 polyester. We modified the technique similarly to Sinha and Richard,[51] in that we do not excise any skin, and double-breast the closure by redraping the fascia flap on the sutures and under the skin flap (**Fig. 1**). In reviewing 435 ears in 227 patients Sinha and Richard[51] identified a 2.6% suture extrusion and 3.7% recurrence rate.[51] Of 6 patients with extrusion, only 1 experienced recurrence when the suture was removed. The investigators calculated 95% confidence intervals, with expected suture extrusion rate between 0.5% and 2.97% and recurrence 2.1% to 5.9%. In a case series of 112 ears, our suture-related complications occurred in 3.6% of ears and recurrence rate was 4.5% (**Figs. 2** and **3**). Recurrence occurred at 1.0 to 5.8 years from surgery.[52] The importance of experience with the technique must be stressed. In a separate series of 118 otoplasties performed with this method by 5 different surgeons, 3 high-volume operators had a recurrence rate of 2.2% to 7.5%, whereas patients of 2 low-volume

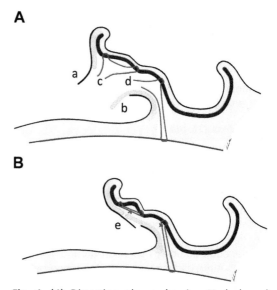

Fig. 1. (*A*) Dissection planes showing Horlock and Gault's dermoepidermal (a) and fascial (b) flaps, and nonabsorbable horizontal mattress sutures positioned to achieve antehelical folding (c) and conchal rotation (d). (*B*) Suturing with Horlock and Gault's flaps closed in double-breasted fashion (e). (*From* Lancerotto L and Stewart KJ. How I do it: Otoplasty. PMFA News 2017;4(3):30. *Reproduced* with kind permission of Pinpoint Scotland Ltd; with permission.)

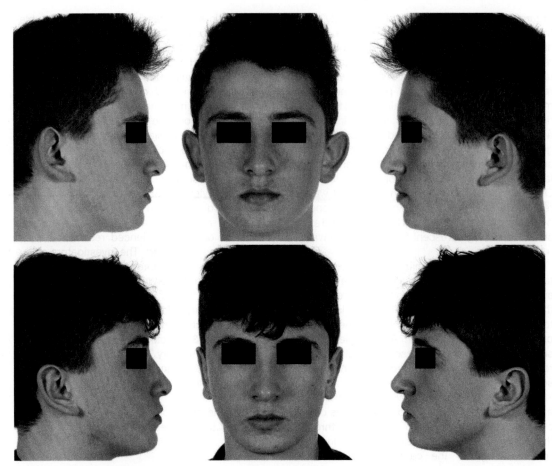

Fig. 2. A case of prominent ears correction by posterior suturing with both antihelical and concho-mastoid sutures, with Horlock and Gault's fascial flap. Top: Preoperative views; bottom: postoperative views.

operators had 50.0% and 66.7% incidence of recurrences.[41]

Incisionless Otoplasty

Peled[53] and Fritsch[54,55] recently proposed a technique of anterior scoring and suturing through minimal percutaneous access, which they called knifeless or incisionless otoplasty. The term is of course a misnomer. Surgery without cutaneous transgression is not possible. The technique is also not completely novel, as the concept of percutaneous suturing has been around for decades.[56] After cartilage scoring, nonabsorbable sutures are inserted via multiple percutaneous passages of the needle and the knots are buried under the postauricular skin. Peled[53] and Haytoglu and colleagues[57] describe a technique for the antihelix, whereas Fritsch[54,55] expands to percutaneous positioning of concho-mastoid and lobe sutures. Very limited reports are available on results. No "significant" complications, such as infection, hematoma, or necrosis, are reported by

any investigator. However, "incisionless" otoplasty seems to encounter a much higher failure and complication rate than more traditional techniques. Combined primary undercorrection and recurrence can be estimated to range between 10% and 25%, and suture complications occur in 12.8% to 26.3% of cases.[57–63] Approximately 2-mm to 3-mm relapse in prominence is to be expected. Failure or recurrence are even higher if reabsorbable sutures are used[53] or cartilage scoring is not performed.[60] In face of this, the advantage of reduced operative times and incidence of anyway rare "major" complications is questionable.

Implants

A recent arrival to the market is the use of gold-plated nickel-titanium alloy superelastic implants.[64] Held straight on a small applicator, these devices are inserted via a small incision within the helical rim. An anterior pocket is created, the implant is released, and reforms to its prebent state. Small

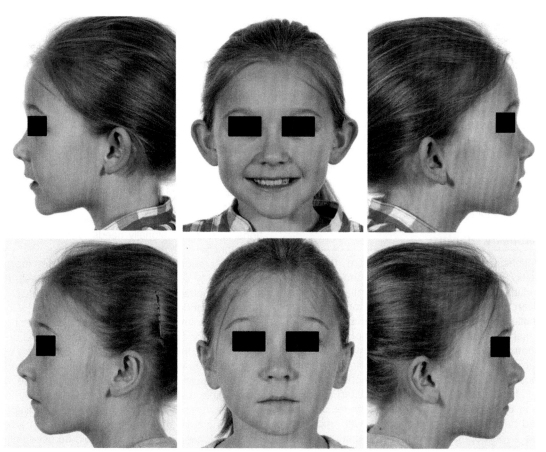

Fig. 3. A second case of otoplasty with the same technique. Top: Preoperative views; bottom: postoperative views.

teeth grip the cartilage and ensure predictable folding. Trial surface devices can be applied with double-sided sticky tape. Thus, a "try before you buy" approach is possible.

These devices offer a quick procedure with predictable outcomes; however, criticism of their use includes implant expense, implant visibility, implant infection risk, extrusion risk, and, finally, much like anterior scoring and "incisionless otoplasty," they rely on overcorrection of the antihelix and fail to properly address the anteriorly rotated conchal bowl. A hidden helix is an all too frequent sequelae. In the only pilot study available, 39 patients were treated. In 21 patients, the implants were removed at 6 to 18 months as part of the study design with prominence recurrence. Recurrence was limited if implants were combined with anterior scoring. Complication incidence was 20.5%, with 5 patients presenting with implant extrusion, 2 cases of implant infection, 2 of hypertrophic scars, and 1 of Spock ear deformity. A significant disadvantage in comparison with suturing techniques is that these adverse events affect the anterior visible surface of the ear.

Comparative Studies

Considering the number of variables in otoplasty techniques, it is no surprise that only a few direct comparative studies are available. Reviews that attempted a comparison of large series recognized this same difficulty, along with the subjectivity in defining success, and the poor documentation of comparable subjective measures.[65] The literature also suffers from publication bias, by which most reports are retrospective, and unfavorable outcomes remain underreported or unreported. Complications with different techniques were reviewed by Limandjaja and colleagues.[44] The extremely wide range of variability for each complication even within theoretically similar techniques likely reflects this issue and hampers the identification of any technique as superior solely based on numbers in comparing studies.

We published 2 studies comparing outcomes with anterior scoring (Chongchet[24]), posterior suturing, and posterior suturing with the Horlock flap within our group.[49,66] In both of these case series, posterior suturing with the Horlock flap emerged as clearly superior to the other 2. It had fewer incidences of both early and late complications. Recurrence rates were 11% and 8% in the first 2 groups, and 4.8% with Horlock's technique. Patient and lay observers rating outcomes as unsatisfactory were again 4 to 5 times less with Horlock and Gault's flap than with Chongchet and traditional Mustardé's procedures. This is at the expense of a relatively longer operative time.[49] Similar results were found in reviewing a smaller cohort of patients who underwent unilateral otoplasty with the same techniques.[66]

Secondary Otoplasty

Unsatisfactory results derive from undercorrections or overcorrections[67] and can imply irreversible distortion of the cartilage frame. Overcorrections and cartilage distortion can be challenging reconstructive problems. At the national referral center for ear reconstruction in Scotland, our group recently reviewed our experience with revision of failed prominent ear corrections.[68] Recurrence of prominence was the dominant cause referral. It accounted for more than 60% of cases in which posterior suturing had been the primary technique, with uncorrected hypertrophic conchal bowl accounting for another 10%. When anterior scoring had been performed, prominence represented in only 38% of referred cases. Only approximately 25% of posterior suturing cases presented with "irreversible" damage requiring major reconstruction, versus more than 60% for anterior scoring cases, of which most consisted of distortion of the scaphoid fossa. Undercorrection/recurrence is approached by diagnosing its origin first, whether in the antehelix, superior crus, concha, or lobule. In most cases, a secondary otoplasty with posterior sutures or conchal cartilage excision yielded satisfactory results. Overcorrection and deformity can require a combination of skin flaps to address an obliterated postauricular sulcus along with cartilage grafts, up to complete ear reconstruction.

Other Techniques

Not all "otoplasty" patients present with prominent ears. Other techniques may be used for alternative indications. Detailed description is beyond our scope. However, ear thinning, ear reduction, and ear augmentation (cartilage grafts) all have a place in the armamentarium of the auricular plastic surgeon.

SUMMARY

It should be noticed that regardless of the technique used, patient satisfaction tends to be high and range above 95%. This is higher than surgeons' opinions on the same cases, which reflects the fact that patients are usually satisfied by having their ears set back, whereas the surgeon better appreciates asymmetries or deformities. This notwithstanding, complications can occur and may be difficult to resolve. Posterior suturing with Horlock and Gault flaps is the technique that when properly performed provides the most immediate control on outcomes. At the same time, it carries less risk of the more serious complications. It very occasionally needs to be combined with conchal resection or cartilage weakening.

Anterior scoring involves higher risk of more serious early and late complications. By itself, it seems to offer no superior protection against recurrence and treats the antihelix alone.

Hybrid techniques combining anterior scoring and posterior suturing may offer minimal recurrence rates. However, they also carry the risks of both techniques. Considering the already limited risk of recurrence with posterior suturing alone, it is advisable that hybridization is reserved only to a very few cases in which the need for cartilage weakening is identified. The same applies to cartilage incision/excision, which should be used only when strictly required.

REFERENCES

1. ASPS. 2016 National Plastic Surgery statistics. 2017. Available at: https://d2wirczt3b6wjm.cloudfront.net/News/Statistics/2016/2016-plastic-surgery-statistics-report.pdf. Accessed April 03, 2017.
2. BAAPS. The bust boom busts. 2017. Available at: http://baaps.org.uk/about-us/press-releases/2366-the-bust-boom-busts. Accessed April 03, 2017.
3. ISAPS. International Survey on Aesthetic/Cosmetic. 2016. Available at: https://www.isaps.org/Media/Default/global-statistics/2016%20ISAPS%20Results.pdf. Accessed April 03, 2017.
4. Matsuo K, Hayashi R, Kiyono M, et al. Nonsurgical correction of congenital auricular deformities. Clin Plast Surg 1990;17:383–95.
5. Smith W, Toye J, Reid A, et al. Nonsurgical correction of congenital ear abnormalities in the newborn: case series. Paediatr Child Health 2005;10:327–31.
6. van Wijk MP, Breugem CC, Kon M. Non-surgical correction of congenital deformities of the auricle: a systematic review of the literature. J Plast Reconstr Aesthet Surg 2009;62:727–36.
7. van Wijk MP, Breugem CC, Kon M. A prospective study on non-surgical correction of protruding

ears: the importance of early treatment. J Plast Reconstr Aesthet Surg 2012;65:54–60.

8. Byrd HS, Langevin CJ, Ghidoni LA. Ear molding in newborn infants with auricular deformities. Plast Reconstr Surg 2010;126:1191–200.

9. Balogh B, Millesi H. Are growth alterations a consequence of surgery for prominent ears? Plast Reconstr Surg 1992;90:192–9.

10. Gosain AK, Kumar A, Huang G. Prominent ears in children younger than 4 years of age: what is the appropriate timing for otoplasty? Plast Reconstr Surg 2004;114:1042–54.

11. Spielmann PM, Harpur RH, Stewart KJ. Timing of otoplasty in children: what age? Eur Arch Otorhinolaryngol 2009;266:941–2.

12. Stewart K, Majdak-Paredes E. Injury patterns and reconstruction in acquired ear deformities. Facial Plast Surg 2015;31:645–56.

13. Wickert N, Wong-Riff K, Mansour M, et al. Developing content for a patient-reported outcome instrument for ear anomalies: a qualitative study. Poster session presented at: 23rd Annual Conference of the International Society of Quality of Life Research. Copenhagen, Denmark. October 19–22, 2016. Qual Life Res 2016;25:1–196.

14. Wang B, Dong Y, Zhao Y, et al. Computed tomography measurement of the auricle in Han population of north China. J Plast Reconstr Aesthet Surg 2011;64:34–40.

15. Rogers BO. The classic reprint. A new operation for prominent ears based on the anatomy of the deformity by William H. Luckett, M.D. (reprinted from Surg. Gynec. & Obst., 10: 635-7, 1910). Plast Reconstr Surg 1969;43:83–6.

16. Erol OO. New modification in otoplasty: anterior approach. Plast Reconstr Surg 2001;107:193–202.

17. Obadia D, Quilichini J, Hunsinger V, et al. Cartilage splitting without stitches: technique and outcomes. JAMA Facial Plast Surg 2013;15:428–33.

18. de la Fuente A, Sordo G. Minimally invasive otoplasty: technical details and long-term results. Aesthetic Plast Surg 2012;36:77–82.

19. Converse JM, Johnson N, Nigro A, et al. A technique for surgical correction of lop ears. Trans Am Acad Ophthalmol Otolaryngol 1956;60:551–6.

20. Converse JM, Wood-Smith D. Technical details in the surgical correction of the lop ear deformity. Plast Reconstr Surg 1963;31:118–28.

21. Baker DC, Converse JM. Correction of protruding ears: a 20-year retrospective. Aesthetic Plast Surg 1979;3:29–39.

22. Gibson T, Davis WB. The distortion of autogenous cartilage grafts: its cause and prevention. Br J Plast Surg 1957;10:257–74.

23. Stenstroem SJ. A "natural" technique for correction of congenitally prominent ears. Plast Reconstr Surg 1963;32:509–18.

24. Chongchet VA. Method of antihelix reconstruction. Br J Plast Surg 1963;16:268–72.

25. Raunig H. Antihelix plasty without modeling sutures. Arch Facial Plast Surg 2005;7:334–41.

26. Vecchione TR. Needle scoring of the anterior surface of the cartilage in otoplasty. Plast Reconstr Surg 1979;64:568.

27. Bulstrode NW, Huang S, Martin DL. Otoplasty by percutaneous anterior scoring. Another twist to the story: a long-term study of 114 patients. Br J Plast Surg 2003;56:145–9.

28. Weinzweig N, Chen L, Sullivan WG. Histomorphology of neochondrogenesis after antihelical fold creation: a comparison of three otoplasty techniques in the rabbit. Ann Plast Surg 1994;33:371–6.

29. Caouette-Laberge L, Guay N, Bortoluzzi P, et al. Otoplasty: anterior scoring technique and results in 500 cases. Plast Reconstr Surg 2000;105:504–15.

30. Calder JC, Naasan A. Morbidity of otoplasty: a review of 562 consecutive cases. Br J Plast Surg 1994;47:170–4.

31. Tolhurst DE. The correction of prominent ears. Br J Plast Surg 1972;25:261–5.

32. Crikelair GF, Cosman B. Another solution for the problem of the prominent ear. Ann Surg 1964;160:314–24.

33. Kaye BL. A simplified method for correcting the prominent ear. Plast Reconstr Surg 1973;52:184.

34. Kompatscher P, Schuler CH, Clemens S, et al. The cartilage-sparing versus the cartilage-cutting technique: a retrospective quality control comparison of the Francesconi and Converse otoplasties. Aesthetic Plast Surg 2003;27:446–53.

35. Eryilmaz T, Ozmen S, Cukurluoglu O, et al. External Mustarde suture technique in otoplasty revisited: a report of 82 cases. J Plast Surg Hand Surg 2013;47:324–7.

36. Irkoren S, Kucukkaya D, Sivrioglu N, et al. Using bilaterally fascioperichondrial flaps with a distal and a proximal base combined with conventional otoplasty. Eur Arch Otorhinolaryngol 2014;271:1389–93.

37. Connolly A, Bartley J. 'External' Mustarde suture technique in otoplasty. Clin Otolaryngol Allied Sci 1998;23:97–9.

38. Mustarde JC. The correction of prominent ears using simple mattress sutures. Br J Plast Surg 1963;16:170–8.

39. Mustarde JC. The treatment of prominent ears by buried mattress sutures: a ten-year survey. Plast Reconstr Surg 1967;39:382–6.

40. Furnas DW. Correction of prominent ears by conchamastoid sutures. Plast Reconstr Surg 1968;42:189–93.

41. Arkoulis N, Reid J, Neill CO, et al. Otoplasty: the case for skin incision by higher volume operators. J Plast Reconstr Aesthet Surg 2015;68:226–9.

42. Davenport G, Bernard FD. Experience with the mattress suture technique in the correction of prominent ears. Plast Reconstr Surg 1965;36:91–6.
43. Maslauskas K, Astrauskas T, Viksraitis S, et al. Comparison of otoplasty outcomes using different types of suture materials. Int Surg 2010;95:88–93.
44. Limandjaja GC, Breugem CC, Mink van der Molen AB, et al. Complications of otoplasty: a literature review. J Plast Reconstr Aesthet Surg 2009;62:19–27.
45. Tan KH. Long-term survey of prominent ear surgery: a comparison of two methods. Br J Plast Surg 1986;39:270–3.
46. Rigg BM. Suture materials in otoplasty. Plast Reconstr Surg 1979;63:409–10.
47. Vuyk HD. Cartilage-sparing otoplasty: a review with long-term results. J Laryngol Otol 1997;111:424–30.
48. Horlock N, Misra A, Gault DT. The postauricular fascial flap as an adjunct to Mustarde and Furnas type otoplasty. Plast Reconstr Surg 2001;108:1487–90.
49. Mandal A, Bahia H, Ahmad T, et al. Comparison of cartilage scoring and cartilage sparing otoplasty–a study of 203 cases. J Plast Reconstr Aesthet Surg 2006;59:1170–6.
50. Basat SO, Ceran F, Askeroglu U, et al. Preventing suture extrusion and recurrence in Mustarde and Furnas otoplasties by using laterally based postauricular dermal flap, long-term results. J Craniofac Surg 2016;27:1476–80.
51. Sinha M, Richard B. Postauricular fascial flap and suture otoplasty: a prospective outcome study of 227 patients. J Plast Reconstr Aesthet Surg 2012;65:367–71.
52. Schaverien MV, Al-Busaidi S, Stewart KJ. Long-term results of posterior suturing with postauricular fascial flap otoplasty. J Plast Reconstr Aesthet Surg 2010;63:1447–51.
53. Peled IJ. Knifeless otoplasty: how simple can it be? Aesthetic Plast Surg 1995;19:253–5.
54. Fritsch MH. Incisionless otoplasty. Laryngoscope 1995;105:1–11.
55. Fritsch MH. Incisionless otoplasty. Otolaryngol Clin North Am 2009;42:1199–208.
56. Kaye BL. A simplified method for correcting the prominent ear. Plast Reconstr Surg 1967;40:44–8.
57. Haytoglu S, Haytoglu TG, Yildirim I, et al. A modification of incisionless otoplasty for correcting the prominent ear deformity. Eur Arch Otorhinolaryngol 2015;272:3425–30.
58. Strychowsky JE, Moitri M, Gupta MK, et al. Incisionless otoplasty: a retrospective review and outcomes analysis. Int J Pediatr Otorhinolaryngol 2013;77:1123–7.
59. Haytoglu S, Haytoglu TG, Bayar Muluk N, et al. Comparison of two incisionless otoplasty techniques for prominent ears in children. Int J Pediatr Otorhinolaryngol 2015;79:504–10.
60. Haytoglu S, Haytoglu TG, Kuran G, et al. Effects of cartilage scoring in correction of prominent ear with incisionless otoplasty technique in pediatric patients. J Int Adv Otol 2016. https://doi.org/10.5152/iao.2016.
61. Ozturan O, Dogan R, Eren SB, et al. Percutaneous adjustable closed otoplasty for prominent ear deformity. J Craniofac Surg 2013;24:398–404.
62. Ozturan O, Dogan R, Eren SB, et al. Cartilage-sparing techniques versus percutaneous adjustable closed otoplasty for prominent ear deformity. J Craniofac Surg 2014;25:752–7.
63. Mehta S, Gantous A. Incisionless otoplasty: a reliable and replicable technique for the correction of prominauris. JAMA Facial Plast Surg 2014;16:414–8.
64. Kang NV, Kerstein RL. Treatment of prominent ears with an implantable clip system: a pilot study. Aesthet Surg J 2016;36:NP100–116.
65. Richards SD, Jebreel A, Capper R. Otoplasty: a review of the surgical techniques. Clin Otolaryngol 2005;30:2–8.
66. Szychta P, Stewart KJ. Comparison of cartilage scoring and cartilage sparing techniques in unilateral otoplasty: a ten-year experience. Ann Plast Surg 2013;71:522–7.
67. Lentz AK, Plikaitis CM, Bauer BS. Understanding the unfavorable result after otoplasty: an integrated approach to correction. Plast Reconstr Surg 2011;128:536–44.
68. Szychta P, Orfaniotis G, Stewart KJ. Revision otoplasty: an algorithm. Plast Reconstr Surg 2012;130:907–16.

Cosmetic Otoplasty

Alexander L. Schneider, MD, Douglas M. Sidle, MD*

KEYWORDS

- Otoplasty • Prominauris • Prominent ear surgery • Mustardé • Furnas

KEY POINTS

- Otoplasty for prominent ears is unique in that it is a widely performed and accepted procedure in the pediatric population, done for cosmetic and not functional motives.
- A detailed knowledge of auricular anatomy and anthropometric norms is essential for the facial plastic surgeon before undertaking any otoplastic surgery.
- There are myriad ways to correct prominauris and the facial plastic surgeon must possess a mastery of a wide variety of techniques to provide durable and acceptable results.

INTRODUCTION

It has been estimated that up to 5% of the population suffers from protruding ears, otherwise known as prominauris.[1] Prominauris is considered to be among the most common congenital deformities of the head and neck region, the most common congenital deformity of the external ear, and is transmitted in autosomal dominant fashion with variable penetrance.[2] This anatomic abnormality typically causes no physiologic change with regards to hearing, though it has rarely in the literature been documented to be an occupational liability in a specific military population.[3] The negative psychosocial impact of prominauris is often the motivating factor to seek surgical correction.[4] In young children and adolescents, the psychological effects are often due to a combination of name-calling, bullying, and ridiculing. The embarrassment and anxiety associated with these psychosocial stressors can lead to increased anxiety, behavioral abnormalities, and result in lack of social integration.[5,6] As a result, otoplasty for the correction of prominauris is a widely accepted cosmetic surgery in the pediatric population that is done solely for aesthetic reasons rather than for correction of an occupational or functional deficit.

EMBRYOLOGY

Before undertaking an intervention to correct prominauris, the surgeon must first possess a comprehensive knowledge of the anatomy of the ear. As with all anatomic knowledge, this begins with understanding the pertinent embryology. The otic placode is the precursor of the ear and develops during the third gestational week. The origin of the auricle (or pinna) is rooted in the concept of the hillocks of His: the hillocks consist of 6 mesodermal swellings that encircle the dorsal surface of the first branchial groove. The first (mandibular) branchial arch is responsible for the development of the 3 cranial-most hillocks, which in turn are responsible for the development of the (1) tragus, (2) helical crus, and (3) helix. The second (hyoid) branchial arch is responsible for the development of the next most caudal hillocks: (4) antihelix, (5) antitragus, and (6) lobule. The hillocks fuse by week 12 and when this fusion occurs inappropriately a preauricular sinus tract may result. The concha is postulated to derive from ectoderm of the first branchial groove, with the upper portion becoming the cymba concha, the middle portion becoming the cavum concha, and the caudal-most portion becoming the intertragal incisura.

Disclosure Statement: The authors have nothing to disclose.
Department of Otolaryngology–Head and Neck Surgery, Northwestern Memorial Hospital, Northwestern University, 676 North Saint Clair, Suite 1325, Chicago, IL 60611, USA
* Corresponding author.
E-mail address: dsidle@nm.org

Facial Plast Surg Clin N Am 26 (2018) 19–29
https://doi.org/10.1016/j.fsc.2017.09.004
1064-7406/18/© 2017 Elsevier Inc. All rights reserved.

SURFACE ANATOMY

The ear is a complex structure composed of elastic cartilage and skin. The 3-dimensional topography of the external ear with its many elevations, depressions, involutions, and folds is reflective of the underlying cartilaginous structure. The auricular cartilage is a single piece of elastic fibrocartilage, invested with perichondrium on all surfaces, and has a relatively uniform thickness throughout. The anterior aspect of the auricle is concave and contains the aforementioned complicated topography, due in large part to the skin envelope of the anterior and lateral auricle being fine, thin, and firmly adherent to the underlying cartilage with little intervening subcutaneous tissue between skin and cartilage. The posterior aspect of the auricle is smooth, convex, and covered with a skin envelope that is considerably less adherent, with a thin subcutaneous areolar tissue layer between the skin and cartilage; these characteristics are useful in flap elevation.

The important surface features of the auricle are seen in **Fig. 1**A. The helix is the peripherally located rim of the auricle. It extends anteriorly to form the root of the helix, or crus of the helix, oriented horizontally above the external acoustic meatus. Immediately inferior to the root of the helix is the tragus. The space between the crus of the helix and the tragus is the anterior incisure. The antitragus is posteroinferior to the tragus, and the space between the tragus and antitragus is known as the intertragal incisure. The antihelix begins at the antitragus and runs anterior and parallel to the helix, initially as a single prominence. In its superior-most extent, the antihelix splits into superior (posterior) and inferior (anterior) crura, and the depression created by this division is known as the triangular fossa. The deep concave furrow in between the helix and the antihelix is known as the scapha or scaphoid fossa. The concha is a cavity posterior to the external auditory meatus and surrounded by the antihelical fold. The crus of the helix divides the conchal cavity into the cymba (superior) and cavum (inferior) concha, which is approximately 8 mm deeper than the tragus and antitragus. Below the antitragus is the lobule, which is devoid of cartilage, composed entirely of areolar connective tissue and fat, and marks an important landmark for the inferior auricle.

NEUROVASCULAR SUPPLY

The neurovascular structures of the auricle are shown in **Fig. 2**A, B. Arterial blood supply to the ear is primarily derived from branches of the external carotid artery, superficial temporal artery (anterior), occipital artery (posterior), and posterior auricular artery (posterior). The superficial temporal artery exits the substance of the parotid gland, travels beneath the anterior auricular muscle, and then divides into branches that supply the anterior auricle. The posterior auricular artery leaves the external carotid artery, runs deep to the posterior auricular muscle and great auricular nerve, and branches to supply the posterior surface of the ear. Venous drainage consists of veins of the same name, which ultimately drain into the external jugular vein. The end branches of these vessels form an extensive anastomotic blood supply to the auricle, which is of great import for local flap auricular reconstruction. The sensory innervation of the external ear is complex. The great auricular nerve, a branch of the cervical plexus, innervates the inferior surface. The lesser occipital, also a branch of the cervical plexus, innervates the posterior superior surface. The auriculotemporal nerve, a branch of the mandibular component of the trigeminal nerve, innervates the anterior superior surface. The concha proper and tragus are innervated by the Arnold nerve, which is a small distal branch of the vagus nerve.

AURICULAR MUSCULATURE

The musculature of the auricle can be divided into extrinsic and intrinsic muscles. The extrinsic muscles connect the auricle with the skull and scalp, whereas the intrinsic connect different parts of the auricle to each other. The superior auricular is the largest of the external muscles. It is thin, fan-shaped, and has its origin on the lateral aspect of the galea aponeurotica, inserting onto the superior aspect of the cranial surface of the auricle. The anterior auricular muscle is also thin and fan-shaped, arises from the anterolateral edge of the galea aponeurotica, and inserts onto a projection on the front of the helix. The posterior auricular consists of 2 to 3 fascicles. It is smaller, has its origin in the mastoid portion of the temporal bone, and inserts onto the inferior aspect of the cranial surface of the concha. The intrinsic auricular muscles are primarily composed of helicis major, helicis minor, tragus, and antitragicus, which surround the conchal bowl. Cranial nerve VII supplies the auricular musculature via its posterior auricular and temporal branches, though these muscles generally have very little volitional movement.

NORMAL ANTHROPOMETRIC FEATURES

Anthropometric studies have revealed that the vertical length of the adult auricle measures between

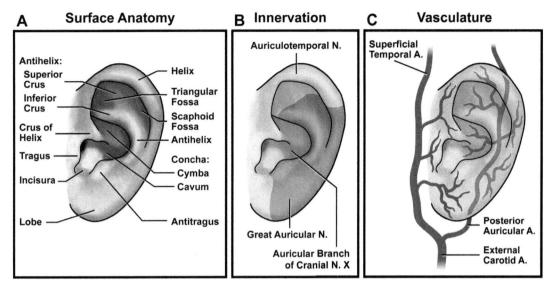

Fig. 1. Topography and neurovascular anatomy of the ear. (*A*) External and topographic landmarks of the external ear. The conchal bowl and antihelix are the most important of external ear landmarks to consider when undertaking cosmetic otoplasty. (*B*) Innervation of the external ear is complex and provided by multiple nerves. (*C*) Vascular supply to the external ear demonstrates the anterior and posterior supply based on branches of the external carotid artery. The superficial temporal artery exits the parotid gland and runs deep to the anterior auricular muscle before dividing into terminal branches that feed the anterior auricle. The posterior auricular artery leaves the external carotid and runs deep to the posterior auricular muscle and great auricular nerve before forming terminal branches that supply the posterior surface of the ear.

approximately 5 cm and 6 cm, and the width should be approximately 55% of its length.[7] Idealized dimensions of the adult ear vary between men and women, with the female ideal dimensions averaging 59.0 mm by 32.5 mm, whereas the ideal male dimensions are 63.5 mm by 35.3 mm. These dimensions is shown in **Fig. 2A**.[8] The external ear develops rapidly at a young age, with 90% of adult width being reached by 1 year of age and between 97% and 99% of adult width being reached by age 10 years. The vertical dimension of the ear develops slower, reaching 75% of adult length by 1 year of age and 93% by age 10 years.[9] Overall, the ear is 85% developed by age 3 years.[10]

The ear should occupy a region corresponding to that from the brow superiorly to the base of

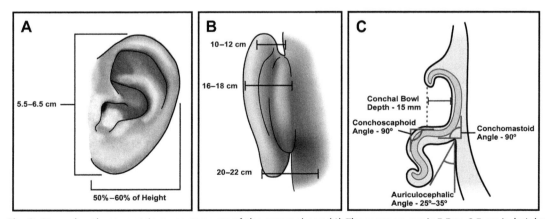

Fig. 2. Normal anthropometric measurements of the external ear. (*A*) The average ear is 5.5 to 6.5 cm in height and the width is 50%-60% of the height. (*B*) Normal measurements from helix to mastoid region are 10 to 12 cm at the superior helix, 16 to 18 cm at the midhelix, and 20 cm to 22 cm at the inferior helix. (*C*) The normal depth of the conchal bowl is less than 1.5 cm. The normal conchomastoid and conchoscaphoid angles are approximately 90°. The normal auriculocephalic angle is between 25° and 35°.

the columella inferiorly and, in the aesthetically pleasing face, the base of the tragus should begin 1 ear width lateral to the lateral canthus.[11] On frontal view, the helix should project 2 mm to 5 mm more lateral than the antihelix.[12] The Frankfort plane, which defines the horizontal plane of the skull and is integral in facial aesthetics, is the horizontal line defined by the superior aspect of the tragus and the inferior orbital rims. The craniocaudad dimension of the ear should roughly parallel the orientation of the dorsum of the nose,[13] and the longest axis of the ear should recline posteriorly at approximately 15° to 30° to the vertical, with the ideal long axis of the normal ear being 20° from the vertical axis of the skull.[14] When viewed in the frontal plane, the lobule should reside in a straight line with the cartilage of the helix[15] and ideally does not project lateral to the upper two-thirds of the ear.[11] Anthropometric studies have revealed important normative measurements discussed in the following section and seen in **Fig. 2**B, C.

The distance between the superior helical rim and mastoid should be between 10 mm and 12 mm, the distance between midhelical rim and mastoid should be between 16 mm and 18 mm, and the distance between the caudal helix and the mastoid should be between 20 mm and 22 mm, as is seen in **Fig. 2**B.[16] The normal ear angulations are seen in **Fig. 2**C and include:

- Conchomastoid angle: The angle at which the conchal bowl rises away from the mastoid cortex. This should be approximately 90°.[17]
- Conchoscaphal angle: This defines the antihelix and should be approximately 90°. More obtuse angles are encountered in patients with prominent ears.
- Auriculocephalic angle: This is the measure of ear projection at the helical root, and is a combination of the preceding 2 angles in combination with the curvature of the helix. In lay terms, it measures how far the pinna sits away from the posterior cranium. This angle is determined by a line extending from the helical root to the most lateral border of the helix and the plane of the mastoid. It should be between 25° and 35°.

PROMINAURIS

Two predominant deformities account for most of the anatomic abnormality in patients with prominauris and, although they may appear individually or in combination, most patients will exhibit some combination of the 2. The more common of the 2 is a poorly developed or unfurled antihelix

that may involve both the superior and inferior crura.[18] Embryologically speaking, the margins of the auricle curl inwards during the sixth fetal month; subsequently, the antihelix folds inward to form the superior and inferior crura, bringing the auricle closer to the head. Thus the lack of an antihelix will cause the ear to be less furled back on itself, the concha will flow directly into the scapha without any clear line of demarcation, and the auricle will protrude further than normal from the head.[18] The second-most common abnormality that causes prominauris is conchal bowl cartilage deformity or excess (>1.5 cm), particularly in the posterior conchal wall.[18,19] The midportion of the helix appears to protrude further when the vertical conchal wall is too high. A conchoscaphal angle greater than 90° also contributes to prominauris because the upper helix will become abnormally anterolaterally displaced and the fossa triangularis will become effaced. An overprojected or protruding lobule also will contribute to prominauris. This anomaly can be present concomitantly with the aforementioned abnormalities or come about as a result of surgery to improve the aforementioned abnormalities.[20] Finally, any skull abnormality may influence the connection of the auricle to the head and influence the appearance of the ear.

OTOPLASTY HISTORY

Techniques for auricular reconstruction have been documented as far back as the seventh century in the writings of Sushruta,[21] a forefather of Ayurveda, in whose ancient scripts modern plastic surgery has roots. In the mid-sixteenth century, Tagliacozzi, an Italian surgeon, published *De Curtorum Chirurgi*, which described methods for auricular reconstruction using postauricular flaps. It was Johann Dieffenbach, a Prussian surgeon, however, who published the first technique for treating prominent ears (of note, however, he was treating a posttraumatic prominent auricle) in which he excised retroauricular skin and used a conchomastoidal suture for fixation of the ear.[22] In 1881, Ely published the first English-language description of otoplasty, in which he took full-thickness excisions of both cartilage and skin via an anterior approach. Even at this early stage, it was seen that full-thickness cartilaginous excisions carried the risk of sharp or unnatural cartilaginous ridging.[23] Morestin, in the early 1900s, described breaking the so-called spring of the conchal cartilage by full-thickness excising of part of its medial wall. In 1910, Luckett described the essential idea of reestablishing the absent antihelical fold to improve on the prominent appearance of the auricle. This was done by excising postauricular skin at the level of the proposed new antihelix and fully excising the cartilage around the new antihelix position to restore the fold and then suturing the edges. Luckett used horizontal mattress sutures to place the flat surfaces (rather than the edges) of the concha and new antihelix in apposition.[24,25] Observing the overcorrected appearance of otoplasty techniques at the time, in 1952, Becker[26] publicized the use of making partial-thickness incisions along the antihelix and then using posterior mattress suture techniques for conical antihelical tubing. Gibson and Davis[27] demonstrated that cartilage injured on 1 side would warp to the opposite side, and this phenomenon formed the basis for many antihelix region incision-scoring techniques moving forward, which used, among other tools, rasps and scalpels. Mustardé, in 1963, introduced the use of only sutures to recreate the antihelical fold, without excising cartilage, as a means of arriving at a natural-appearing antihelix.[28] The conchomastoid setback, perhaps better known as the Furnas technique, was described in 1968 by Furnas[29] and in 1969 by Spira and colleagues.[30]

OTOPLASTY FOR PROMINAURIS TECHNIQUES: CARTILAGE-CUTTING VERSUS CARTILAGE-SPARING

Otoplasty operations are individually tailored to each patient; however, the classic goals of otoplasty were outlined in 1968 by McDowell[31] and hold true to this day:

1. All upper third ear protrusion must be corrected
2. The helix of both ears should be seen beyond the antihelix from the front view
3. The helix should have a smooth and regular line throughout
4. The postauricular sulcus should not be markedly decreased or distorted
5. The helix to mastoid distance should be in the normal range of 10 mm to 12 mm in the upper third, 16 mm to 18 mm in the middle third, and 20 mm to 22 mm in the lower third
6. The position of the lateral ear border to the head should match within 3 mm at any point between the 2 ears.

Hundreds of techniques have been described for the correction of prominauris since the inception of cosmetic otoplasty and, though hotly debated, no single approach has become universally favored. Otoplasty techniques have been typically divided into 2 overarching divisions: cartilage cutting and cartilage reshaping or sparing, including solely cartilage suturing. Cartilage-cutting techniques include scoring, abrading, excising, and making full-thickness or partial-thickness incisions into the auricular cartilage. These procedures depend on cartilage bending away from the cut side and, typically, have been thought to improve the duration of surgical results, though there is clearly an increased risk of postoperative cosmetic deformity secondary to the sharp surfaces created when cartilage is cut to any degree. Purely cartilage-reshaping technique implies using only sutures to recreate normal auricular anatomy. Scarring, as well as the aforementioned contour deformities, is largely avoided with suture-only otoplasty; however, there is a higher rate of persistent or recurrent auricular abnormality.

Regardless of the technique, before surgery a comprehensive preoperative history and physical should be performed. Protrusion, proportionality to facial structures and head, angular relationships of mastoid to auricle and concha, and all other deformities should be noted for each ear individually and in relation to each other. With all cosmetic procedures, preoperative and postoperative photographs are essential for planning and documentation purposes. The following views are recommended: full-head posterior, full-facial frontal, bilateral close-up of each ear, and oblique shots of each ear. A craniocaudal photograph may be used for assessing lateral auricular projection. The hair should be swept away from the ears with the patient's preferred method, which may be headband or hairclip. Photographs should be taken in the Frankfort plane when possible, and uniform lighting should be used for both preoperative and postoperative photographs. An assessment of the patient (and often of the patient's parents) is also important. An understanding of the patient's goals for the operation should be attained, and realistic expectations should be ensured in this regard. Complications and the importance of adhering to postoperative instructions should also be discussed in detail with the patient and/or parents.

CARTILAGE-CUTTING OTOPLASTY

In the category of cartilage-cutting otoplasty, 1 of the best known early techniques on which subsequent techniques are based was put forth by Converse and colleagues[32] in 1955. This method is intended to recreate the antihelical fold. The original Converse technique involved the following steps: (1) folding back the ear until a normal antihelix curvature is seen and then outlining the limits of the new antihelix, (2) excising an ellipse of skin from the posterior auricle, (3) making full-thickness incisions through the outlined cartilage,

(4) folding back and tubing the incised segment to create the appearance of an antihelix, and (5) securing the tube with sutures to create a new antihelical fold. The cartilage-cutting method of Davis addresses conchal bowl hypertrophy in a way that some investigators have postulated to provide longer lasting effects than the cartilage-sparing methods of altering conchal bowl hypertrophy.[33]

In the Davis procedure, a calipers is used to define at least 8 mm to 10 mm of conchal wall and bowl that will remain intact. Methylene blue-tipped hypodermic needles are used to make transcartilaginous tattoos through and through the conchal bowl such that the surgeon can see her or his markings on the posterior conchal cartilage. Similar to the Furnas method, the soft tissue in the postauricular region is removed down to the level of the mastoid fascia. Then the posterior concha is found via an elliptical postauricular skin excision, making sure that the planned incision is large enough to remove the excess skin after the cartilage is removed. At this point, a kidney bean–shaped portion of cartilage should be outlined by the transcartilaginous blue needle dots, and the surgeon sharply carries dissection through the marks, being careful not to penetrate the anterior dermal surface of the conchal bowl skin. Finally, the excess cartilage is removed and the ear should be passively laid posteriorly to assess if any further resection is required. The postauricular incision is closed. Bolstering sutures can be placed through the ear, into the exposed mastoid fascia, back through the ear, and tied down through dental rolls. Alternatively, the mastoid fascia and the posterior conchal wall may be secured directly with absorbable suture and the surgeon's bolster of choice may be placed.[10,33]

CARTILAGE-SPARING OTOPLASTY

The cartilage-sparing techniques have the advantages of maintaining the cartilage's natural contour as the cartilage itself is never cut or incised. Also, they are easier to adjust intraoperatively, given that stitches can be tightened to assess results before tying them. The primary disadvantage of the cartilage-sparing otoplasty techniques is that, in the face of stiff auricular cartilage, they are more likely to result in recurrent deformity. Thus cartilage-sparing otoplasty is more likely to allow for durable results in the pediatric patient population. Two of the most well-known cartilage-sparing otoplasty techniques are the Mustardé and the Furnas (conchal setback).

The primary objective of the Mustardé otoplasty is to recreate the antihelix using sutures only,

reshaping the cartilage without directly incising it. To do this, the helical rim is posteriorly displaced using the surgeon's finger until an appropriately sized antihelix is seen. The midline of the antihelical fold should be marked and planned suture points similarly marked out, at a distance of 7 mm to 8 mm from the midline on both sides of the midline of the antihelical fold. Once prepped, draped, and anesthetized, the authors' typically use 27-gauge needles dipped in methylene blue to go through and through the auricular cartilage at each of the planned entry points that should be 7 mm to 8 mm from the midline of the antihelical fold. The planned antihelix is shown in **Figs. 3**A and **4**A. An elliptical postauricular skin incision is then executed with a number 15 blade. It is the authors' practice to carry out a W-plasty at the superior aspect of the incision, as is shown in **Fig. 4**B, to better excise the excess skin. From this point forward, sharp dissection is carried out with curved iris scissors, and the subperichondrial dissection is carried out after resecting the skin involved with the incision and the underlying subcutaneous tissue. Anywhere from 3 to 4 horizontal mattress sutures are placed through the tattooed dots, using nonabsorbable clear or transparent sutures, going through the auricular cartilage and perichondrium but not through the anterior skin of the auricle. **Fig. 4**C demonstrates the intraoperative view of the needle dipped in methylene blue having gone through and through the cartilage, marking the points for horizontal mattress Mustardé sutures. The ear should be periodically turned over to verify that the skin has not been pierced. The stitches may be secured with a hemostat and the resultant antihelical fold should be visualized before tying the stitches. The order in which the stitches are tied varies in the literature. Some surgeons tie from superior to inferior, whereas others tie the middle stitch first, then the inferior, and finally the superior. The process of tying each Mustardé stitch is shown in a representative illustration in **Fig. 3**B and a cross-sectional representation of a completely tied down stitch is demonstrated in **Fig. 3**C. The incision is then closed with interrupted buried absorbable suture, followed by running fast-absorbing suture, leaving a small opening at the inferior aspect of the incision for any drainage.

The technique originally described by Furnas[29] in 1968 deals with the second-most common auricular deformity responsible for prominauris, the abnormally enlarged conchal bowl, in a cartilage-sparing manner. This should be performed before correcting the deficient antihelix because, once the conchal bowl has been set back, the need to correct the deficient antihelix

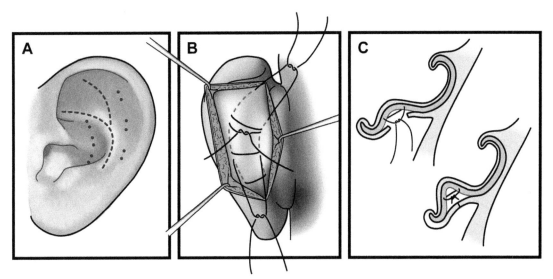

Fig. 3. Mustardé technique. (*A*) The midline of the planned antihelical fold is marked with a marking pen before making an incision and dots are made in the locations of the planned Mustardé horizontal mattress stitches. (*B*) The horizontal mattress stitches used to create the antihelical fold are demonstrated, with each being half-tied before the final knots are thrown. (*C*) Cross-sectional demonstration of Mustardé sutures with the incision closed.

will have often been ameliorated.[34] The surgeon's small instrument of choice (eg, cotton-tipped applicator) is used to press the conchal bowl against the mastoid to the point that the ear is no longer prominent. The meeting of the 2 surfaces is marked in the conchal bowl. An elliptical area of postauricular skin is removed to expose the posterior surface of the auricular cartilage, removing the posterior auricular muscles and ligaments but saving any branches of the great auricular nerve. Then, an approximately 1 cm by 2 cm area of deep mastoid fascia is exposed; 4-0 nonabsorbable sutures are passed into the mastoid periosteum, full-thickness through and through the cartilage (without perforating the anterior conchal skin), and back into the periosteum. Typically, 2 to 3 are placed and half-tightened to assess effect before tying the final knots. The process of tying the knots and a representative Furnas

conchomastoid setback is shown in **Fig. 5**. Care must be taken with placement because it is well documented that sutures placed too far anteriorly on the mastoid or posteriorly on the conchal cartilage have the potential to exaggerate the anterior or posterior rotation of the ear and may cause narrowing of the external auditory canal.[35] Finally, the incision is closed with buried absorbable braided sutures followed by running fast-absorbing suture, leaving a small opening at the inferior aspect of the incision for drainage. The preoperative and postoperative view of a teenage patient who underwent both Mustardé and Furnas technique otoplasty is shown in **Fig. 6**.

LOBULE MANAGEMENT

An overprojected or protruding lobule, although not 1 of the 2 classically taught causes of

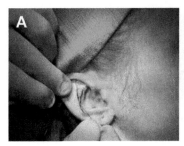
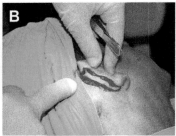
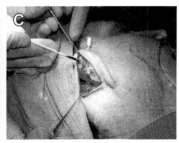

Fig. 4. (*A*) The planned antihelix is marked out anteriorly before making an incision. (*B*) The postauricular incision is completed, including the authors' preferred W-plasty at the superior aspect of the incision. (*C*) Intraoperative view of the needle dipped in methylene blue having gone through and through the cartilage, marking the points for horizontal mattress Mustardé sutures.

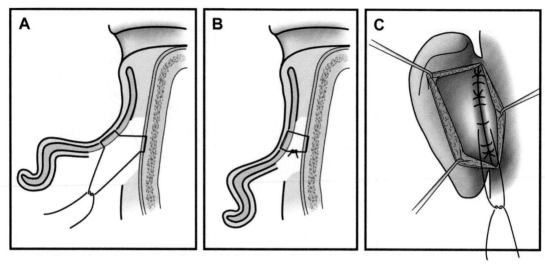

Fig. 5. (*A*) Demonstration of conchomastoid suture before knot being securely tied down. (*B*) Cross-sectional demonstration of conchomastoid setback suture after being securely tied down. (*C*) Demonstration of multiple securely tied conchomastoid sutures before closing the skin incision.

prominauris, plays a role in the prominent ear yet is an often overlooked component of said cosmetic deformity.[10,15] The ideal lobule lies in the same plane vertically as the helix, and a lobule-mastoid angle greater than 40° has been documented as excessive.[36] It has been postulated that even if the lobule is not abnormal at baseline it may ultimately protrude or overproject after otoplastic

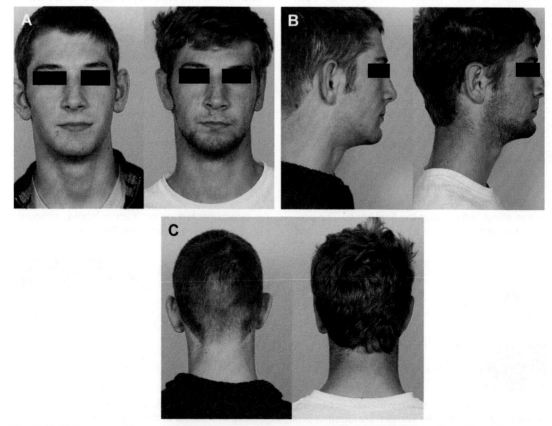

Fig. 6. (*A–C*) Anterior, oblique, and posterior views of a teenage patient with prominauris on the right greater than left, both before and after combined Furnas and Mustardé technique otoplasty.

procedures to address the more cephalic compo-nents of the auricle.[37]

The lobule is thus typically approached after first addressing the other anatomic abnormalities responsible for the patient's prominauris.[38] Though not as frequently published on as methods of conchomastoid setback or antiheli-cal creation, multiple methods of lobule correc-tion have been proposed. One of the more common theories of causes for lobular promi-nence is that of excess lobular skin and fibrofatty tissue.[39] As such, skin excisions have been pro-posed in various forms.[40,41] Typically, the sur-geon will extend the postauricular skin incision inferiorly onto the lobule and then excise skin and underlying fibrofatty tissue. The shape of skin incisions has been described in various ways, including fish-tail, V-shape, and M-plasty.[11,13,22] Spira[42] proposed eccentrically excising posterior lobule skin and then passing a nonabsorbable suture from the lateral dermal aspect of the excised skin to the conchal carti-lage near the mastoid periosteum. Gosain and Recinos[43] proposed a similar procedure but anchored the suture to the mastoid periosteum. Another common theory to explain the protrud-ing lobule is based on the premise that lobule position is controlled by the position of the caudal helix, which is attached to the cephalic aspect of the lobule, relative to the conchal bowl.[37] With this relationship in mind, one can understand the reasoning behind the procedure popularized by Goulian and Conway[44] in which the helix and concha are dissected apart and then the caudal helix is affixed to the concha, in turn altering the position of the lobule.

To conclude, management of the lobule in cosmetic otoplasty can be easily overshadowed by management of the more cephalic anatomic causes of prominauris. Despite being less studied than those causes, the surgeon has multiple ap-proaches to the lobule available. The lower pole of the ear should be scrutinized for asymmetry and overprojection before surgery begins and especially after the upper two-thirds of the ear have been addressedbecause an otherwise perfectly undertaken otoplasty will still yield poor results if the caudal ear is neglected.

COMPLICATIONS

The literature has shown that both pediatric and adult patients benefit psychosocially and emotion-ally after otoplasty surgery.[5,45] The combination of proper preoperative counseling and postoperative alleviation of significant psychosocial distress and anxiety results in a patient population that gener-ally is pleased with their postoperative result.[13,46] The early complications of otoplasty include he-matoma, infection (typically caused by pseudo-monas), and cartilage or skin necrosis.[47] Delayed complications include suture extrusion, scarring, persistent or new asymmetries, and aesthetic complications.[48] Loss of correction is a complica-tion that occurs usually within the first 3 months postoperatively, and may be a result of improper or insufficient amount of suture placement, overly stiff cartilage, a trauma to the ear,[49] or some com-bination of these.

The aesthetic complications of otoplasty vary and, frequently, the surgeon will be more critical of otoplastic aesthetic complications than pa-tients.[50] Common unsatisfactory aesthetic out-comes include the telephone-ear deformity; the reverse telephone-ear deformity; the vertical post deformity; hidden-helix (overcorrection) deformity; and, finally, the appearance of antihelical ridges.

The telephone-ear occurs when there has been overcorrection of the middle vertical third of the ear, as in the case of excess conchal setback or removal of too much postauricular skin in the mid-dle vertical third of the auricle.[51] It conceptually follows that if there is undercorrection of the supe-rior auricle and lobule, the telephone-ear deformity may manifest itself.[48] In these situations, the supe-rior auricle and inferior pole (lobule) may overpro-trude. Treatment may include redoing the Mustardé and/or Furnas sutures to improve the antihelix and conchal position, respectively. In addition, if the lobule has not been deprojected, this would be done as well.[52]

The reverse telephone-ear deformity is the opposite, wherein the middle third is prominent with respect to the superior and inferior poles. This may occur due to failure to address midcon-chal wall height and overcorrection of the superior and inferior poles.[47] One method of treating a reverse telephone-ear deformity is to reperform the conchomastoid stitch.[52]

The vertical post deformity describes the crea-tion of an aberrant superior crus of the antihelix such that the superior crus is oriented in a vertical direction as opposed to the gentle arc as should be seen in a normal helix. This happens when Mustardé sutures are placed in a vertical, as opposed to an oblique, direction.[47,51]

The hidden helix deformity is present in those cases in which there has been an overcorrection of the auricular lateral projection, resulting in the antihelix being the most lateral structure seen on frontal view and the auricle having an overall plastered-down appearance. Two methods to avoid this particular deformity have been postulated to include tying the middle of the Mustardé sutures last, as well as ascertaining the required degree of antihelical creation only after setting back the concha.[53]

Finally, as previously mentioned, pure cartilage-cutting otoplastic techniques pose the risk of eventual visibility of sharp cartilaginous edges or ridges, particularly in the area of the antihelix. One way to prevent this complication is to simply avoid full-thickness cartilage-cutting incisions when recreating the antihelix. When they do become apparent, these sharp edges can be approached in a variety of ways, ranging from using a curette to smooth over small edges, as proposed by Walter and Nolst Trenite[54]; using a small diamond drill to smooth sharp borders[55]; and/or placing temporalis fascia or conchal cartilage grafts into subcutaneous pockets overlying particularly sharp edges.[53] Some publications have noted that the improvement with the latter technique is short-lasting.[56] As with all cosmetic surgery, a thorough informed consent process and addressing unrealistic expectations preoperatively is essential; patients should be counseled that improvement but not perfection is the end goal.

SUMMARY

Prominauris almost never causes an audiological or occupational deficit, yet the mental and emotional strain can take a tremendous negative toll on patients. Otoplasty for prominent ears requires an in-depth knowledge of normal anatomy, embryology, and anthropometric measurements. Though often rewarding for both surgeon and patient, no single technique or procedure will correct prominauris all of the time, and facial plastic surgeons must familiarize themselves with a variety of options to achieve long-lasting and acceptable results.

REFERENCES

1. Salgarello M, Gasperoni C, Montagnese A, et al. Otoplasty for prominent ears: A versatile combined technique to master the shape of the ear. Otolaryngol Head Neck Surg 2007;137(2):224–7.
2. Emery BE. Otoplasty. Facial Plast Surg Clin North Am 2001;9(1):147–57.
3. Salgado CJ, Mardini S. Corrective otoplasty for symptomatic prominent ears in U.S. soldiers. Mil Med 2006;171(2):128–30.
4. Horlock N, Vögelin E, Bradbury ET, et al. Psychosocial outcome of patients after ear reconstruction: a retrospective study of 62 patients. Ann Plast Surg 2005;54(5):517–24.
5. Cooper-Hobson G, Jaffe W. The benefits of otoplasty for children: further evidence to satisfy the modern NHS. J Plast Reconstr Aesthet Surg 2009;62(2):190–4.
6. Songu M, Kutlu A. Health-related quality of life outcome of children with prominent ears after otoplasty. Eur Arch Otorhinolaryngol 2014;271(6):1829–32.
7. Petersson RS, Friedman O. Current trends in otoplasty. Curr Opin Otolaryngol Head Neck Surg 2008;16(4):352–8.
8. Farkas LG. Anthropometry of the normal and defective ear. Clin Plast Surg 1990;17(2):213–21.
9. Janis JE, Rohrich RJ, Gutowski KA. Otoplasty. Plast Reconstr Surg 2005;115(4):60e–72e.
10. Owsley TG. Otoplastic surgery for the protruding ear. Atlas Oral Maxillofac Surg Clin North Am 2004;12(1):131–9.
11. Kelley P, Hollier L, Stal S. Otoplasty: evaluation, technique, and review. J Craniofac Surg 2003;14(5):643–53.
12. Niamtu J. Cosmetic otoplasty and related ear conditions. In: Niamtu J, editor. Cosmetic facial surgery. Saint Louis (MI): Elsevier Mosby; 2011. p. 434–516.
13. Mobley SR, John Vartanian A, Toriumi DM. Otoplasty: surgical correction of the protruding ear. Oper Tech Otolayngol Head Neck Surg 2002;13(1):29–35.
14. Stal S, Klebuc M, Spira M. An algorithm for otoplasty. Oper Tech Otolayngol Head Neck Surg 1997;4(3):88–103.
15. Nuara MJ, Mobley SR. Nuances of otoplasty: a comprehensive review of the past 20 years. Facial Plast Surg Clin North Am 2006;14(2):89–102, vi.
16. Adamson JE, Horton CE, Crawford HH. The growth pattern of the external ear. Plast Reconstr Surg 1965;36(4):466–70.
17. Sclafani A. Otoplasty. In: Sataloff RT, Sclafani AP, Spalla TC, editors. Facial plastic and reconstructive surgery (surgical techniques in otolaryngology head and neck surgery). New Delhi (India): Jaypee Brothers; 2014. p. 113–8.
18. Becker DG, Lai SS, Wise JB, et al. Analysis in otoplasty. Facial Plast Surg Clin North Am 2006;14(2):63–71, v.
19. Perez C. Otoplasty. In: Wong BJ, Arnold MG, Boeckmann JO, editors. Facial plastic and reconstructive surgery: a comprehensive study guide. Switzerland: Springer; 2016. p. 197–208.
20. Rubino C, Farace F, Mulas P. Otoplasty. In: Scuderi N, Toth BA, editors. International textbook of aesthetic surgery. Berlin: Springer; 2016. p. 821–37.
21. Hauben DJ. Sushruta Samhita (Sushruta'a collection) (800-600 B.C.?). Pioneers of plastic surgery. Acta Chir Plast 1984;26(2):65–8.
22. Naumann A. Otoplasty - techniques, characteristics and risks. GMS Curr Top Otorhinolaryngol Head Neck Surg 2007;6:Doc04.

23. Ely E. An operation for prominence of the auricles. Arch Otolaryngol 1881;19:9–99.

24. Rogers BO. The classic reprint. A new operation for prominent ears based on the anatomy of the deformity by William H. Luckett, M.D. (reprinted from Surg. Gynec. & Obst., 10: 635-7, 1910). Plast Reconstr Surg 1969;43(1):83–6.

25. Shiffman MA. History of otoplasty: review of literature. In: Shiffman M, editor. Advanced cosmetic otoplasty: art, science, and new clinical techniques. Berlin: Springer; 2013. p. 43–64.

26. Becker OJ. Correction of the protruding deformed ear. Br J Plast Surg 1952;5(3):187–96.

27. Gibson T, Davis WB. The distortion of autogenous cartilage grafts: Its cause and prevention. Br J Plast Surg 1957;10:257–74.

28. Mustarde JC. The correction of prominent ears using simple mattress sutures. Br J Plast Surg 1963;16:170–8.

29. Furnas DW. Correction of prominent ears by concha-mastoid sutures. Plast Reconstr Surg 1968;42(3):189–93.

30. Spira M, McCrea R, Gerow FJ, et al. Correction of the principal deformities causing protruding ears. Plast Reconstr Surg 1969;44(2):150–4.

31. McDowell AJ. Goals in otoplasty for protruding ears. Plast Reconstr Surg 1968;41(1):17–27.

32. Converse JM, Johnson N, Nigro A, et al. A technique for surgical correction of lop ears. Trans Am Acad Ophthalmol Otolaryngol 1956;60(4):551–6.

33. Niamtu J. Cosmetic otoplasty. Am J Cosmet Surg 2011;28(4):261–72.

34. Ambro BT, Lebeau J. Pediatric otoplasty. Oper Tech Otolaryngol Head Neck Surg 2009;20(3):206–9.

35. Pawar SS, Koch CA, Murakami C. Treatment of prominent ears and otoplasty: a contemporary review. JAMA Facial Plast Surg 2015;17(6):449–54.

36. Michael Sadove A, Eppley BL. Lobule repositioning in aesthetic otoplasty. Oper Tech Plas Recons Surg 1997;4(3):129–33.

37. Isac C, Isac A. Correction of the Protruding Lobule. In: Shiffman M, editor. Advanced cosmetic otoplasty: art, science, and new clinical techniques. Berlin: Springer; 2013. p. 477–80.

38. Bilkay U, Tiftikcioglu YO, Kapi E, et al. Y-to-V setback for prominent lobule correction in otoplasty. Ann Plast Surg 2011;66(6):623–6.

39. Adamson PA, Litner JA. Adjunctive procedures management of the helix scapha and lobule. In: Adamson PA, Litner JA, Thomas RJ, editors. Aesthetic otoplasty: thomas procedures in facial plastic surgery. Shelton (CT): People's Medical Publishing House; 2011. p. 45–54.

40. Lavy J, Stearns M. Otoplasty: techniques, results and complications–a review. Clin Otolaryngol Allied Sci 1997;22(5):390–3.

41. Karagoz H, Eren F, Ulkur E. A new skin excision pattern to correct protruding earlobe deformity in prominent ears. Aesthetic Plast Surg 2012;36(1):215–7.

42. Spira M. Otoplasty: what I do now–a 30-year perspective. Plast Reconstr Surg 1999;104(3):834–40 [discussion: 841].

43. Gosain AK, Recinos RF. A novel approach to correction of the prominent lobule during otoplasty. Plast Reconstr Surg 2003;112(2):575–83.

44. Goulian D Jr, Conway H. Prevention of persistent deformity of the tragus and lobule by modification of the Luckett technique of otoplasty. Plast Reconstr Surg Transplant Bull 1960;26:399–404.

45. Schwentner I, Schmutzhard J, Deibl M, et al. Health-related quality of life outcome of adult patients after otoplasty. J Craniofac Surg 2006;17(4):629–35.

46. Caouette-Laberge L, Guay N, Bortoluzzi P, et al. Otoplasty: anterior scoring technique and results in 500 cases. Plast Reconstr Surg 2000;105(2):504–15.

47. Handler EB, Song T, Shih C. Complications of otoplasty. Facial Plast Surg Clin North Am 2013;21(4):653–62.

48. Limandjaja GC, Breugem CC, Mink van der Molen AB, et al. Complications of otoplasty: a literature review. J Plast Reconstr Aesthet Surg 2009;62(1):19–27.

49. Adamson PA, McGraw BL, Tropper GJ. Otoplasty: critical review of clinical results. Laryngoscope 1991;101(8):883–8.

50. Richards SD, Jebreel A, Capper R. Otoplasty: a review of the surgical techniques. Clin Otolaryngol 2005;30(1):2–8.

51. Sands NB, Adamson PA. Pediatric esthetic otoplasty. Facial Plast Surg Clin North Am 2014;22(4):611–21.

52. Shiffman MA. Otoplasty complications 2013. p. 523–6.

53. Adamson PA, Litner JA. Aesthetic pitfalls in otoplasty. In: Adamson PA, Litner JA, Thomas RJ, editors. Aesthetic otoplasty: Thomas procedures in facial plastic surgery. Shelton (CT): People's Medical Publishing House; 2011. p. 135–46.

54. Walter C, Nolst Trenite GJ. Revision otoplasty and special problems. Facial Plast Surg 1994;10(3):298–308.

55. Freitas RDS, Ono MCC, Alonso N. Solving sharp edges of the antihelix after otoplasty. Berlin: Springer; 2013. p. 535–7.

56. Berghaus A, Braun T, Hempel JM. Revision otoplasty: how to manage the disastrous result. Arch Facial Plast Surg 2012;14(3):205–10.

Otoplasty for Congenital Auricular Malformations

Jiahui Lin, MD[a,b], Anthony P. Sclafani, MD[b,*]

KEYWORDS

- Congenital auricular anomaly • Cryptotia • Stahl ear • Constricted ear • Satyr ear • Lop ear
- Cup ear • Macrotia

KEY POINTS

- Aside from microtia and simple prominent ears, congenital auricular deformities include cryptotia, Stahl ear, constricted ear, and macrotia.
- Congenital auricular deformities are uncommon, and most occur sporadically without association with other anomalies.
- There are as many techniques to surgical correction of congenital auricular anomalies as there are variations of each.

INTRODUCTION

Congenital auricular anomalies are uncommon, with an incidence ranging from 0.8 to 2.4 per 10,000 live births.[1] These anomalies vary in rarity between racial groups, affecting Hispanic, Asian, and Navajo Indian individuals more than European and black individuals.[2]

Congenital auricular anomalies include microtia and prominent ears, and, less commonly, cryptotia, Stahl ear, constricted ear, and macrotia. When evaluating patients for otoplasty, consideration must be made regarding not only the general category of anomaly, but also any variations or combinations of defects that may influence the technique that will be used for repair.

Evaluation of these deformities includes comparing the deformity with the rest of the ear, the abnormal ear with the other side, and its relationship with the rest of the face. The average height and width of the adult ear is 58 mm and 34 mm for women, and 62 mm and 36 mm for men, respectively.[3] The ear also normally protrudes by 17 to 21 mm from the mastoid.[4] Clinicians should use these averages as a guide, rather than strictly adhering to specific measurements.

Auricular anomalies may be secondary to embryologic maldevelopment and/or deformational forces applied either in utero or ex utero.[5] The auricle is embryologically developed from the first (mandibular) and second (hyoid) branchial arches.[3] Because these arches give rise to other parts of the face, some auricular anomalies are sometimes associated with other craniofacial anomalies that form recognized syndromes or sequences, such as Treacher Collins.[5] However, most auricular anomalies occur sporadically. The auricular muscles also have been implicated in auricular anomalies, such as Stahl ear, prominent ears, and cryptotia, as they help determine normal auricular shape.[6–10]

CRYPTOTIA

Cryptotia occurs when the upper pole of the auricle is buried under the temporal skin, leading to an absent sulcus (**Fig. 1**).[11] Cryptotia may be caused by deforming forces from aberrant auricular muscle insertion and may be categorized depending on which muscle is involved (**Box 1**).[5,9] The most common abnormalities have been found in the superior auricular muscle, auricular oblique muscle, and

Disclosure: J. Lin and A.P. Sclafani have nothing they wish to disclose.
[a] Department of Otolaryngology, Columbia University Medical Center, 180 Fort Washington Avenue, New York, NY 10032, USA; [b] Department of Otolaryngology, Weill Cornell Medical College, 1305 York Avenue, New York, NY 10021, USA
* Corresponding author.
E-mail address: ans9243@med.cornell.edu

Facial Plast Surg Clin N Am 26 (2018) 31–40
https://doi.org/10.1016/j.fsc.2017.09.003
1064-7406/18/© 2017 Elsevier Inc. All rights reserved.

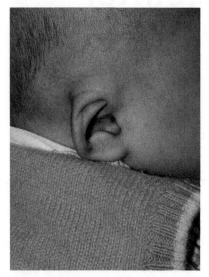

Fig. 1. Cryptotia of the superior pole of the auricle.

transverse auricular muscle.[10,12,13] Many cases involve more than one contributing muscle.

STAHL EAR

Stahl ear is an auricular anomaly that causes the top of the ear to appear pointed and flattened (**Fig. 2**). Specifically, this is caused by hypoplasia of the superior crus of the antihelix, enlargement of the base of the antihelix, as well as development of an extra third crus of the antihelix that connects the antihelix with the posterosuperior part of the helix.[14,15] It is likely that this deformity is a result of dysgenesis of the auricular transverse muscle during embryogenesis, which leads to hypoplasia of the superior crus of the antihelix and the development of the third crus.[6,12,16] Abnormalities in the superior auricular muscle and auricular oblique muscle have also been documented.

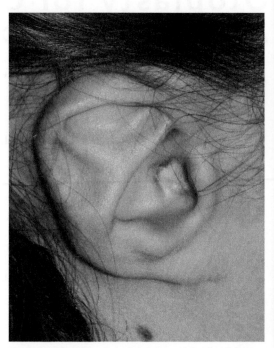

Fig. 2. Stahl deformity of the ear.

Stahl ear has been postulated to have a genetic component of transmission, although this has not been definitively shown.[16] In most cases, Stahl ear occurs sporadically, although one case has been reported in association with Finlay-Marks syndrome, a rare autosomal dominant disorder with anomalies of the scalp, ears, and nipples.[17] Stahl ear is not typically associated with hearing defects.

CONSTRICTED EAR/CUP EAR/LOP EAR/SATYR EAR

Cup ear refers to ear protrusion, and lop ear to an ear with an overhanging upper pole, both of which are often grouped together under the term constricted ear (**Figs. 3** and **4**).[18] Traditionally, constricted ears have been classified using a system first proposed

---

Box 1
Cryptotia classification

- Type I: abnormality of the transverse auricular muscle

  o Compression of the body and superior crus of the antihelix

  o Burying of the upper auricle underneath the skin

- Type II: abnormality of the auricular oblique muscle

  o Gross contraction of the antihelical body

  o Acute bend of the inferior crus of the antihelix

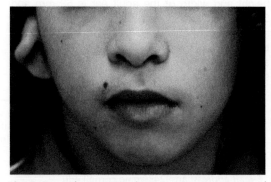

Fig. 3. Severely constricted cup ear. Notice associated hemifacial microsomia.

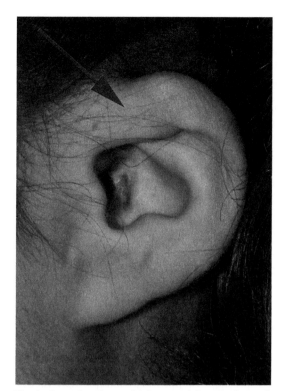

Fig. 4. Constricted ear with lop ear deformity (*arrow*).

superior helix. Abnormalities in the auricular transverse muscle, particularly elongation of the muscle, have been documented in patients with lop ear.[12] This leads to the incorrect folding or creation of the antihelix. Others have also shown that the absence of the posterior auricular muscle may also contribute to lop ear.[23]

Lop ear is sometimes a component of Finlay-Marks syndrome as well (see previously, Stahl ear), and it has been shown to be passed down in an autosomal dominant fashion in some families.[24,25] Satyr ear, a form of lop ear, is associated with Townes-Brocks syndrome, an autosomal dominant disorder with imperforate anus, finger and toe anomalies, and sensorineural hearing loss.[26,27] However, most cases of isolated lop ear are sporadic cases.

MACROTIA

Macrotia is an enlargement of the pinna in length or width.[28] However, when taken in proportion with the rest of the face, the ear as a whole may appear large if its overall length exceeds the middle third of the face.[29] Most commonly, the upper third of the auricle is involved in macrotia, and it is often a component of prominent or protruding ears.[30]

by Tanzer, although a newer system has been introduced by Daniali and colleagues (**Box 2**).[18,19]

Lop ear refers to an abnormal overfolding of the auricle, reduced or absent superior antihelical crus, reduced scapha, reduced fossa triangularis, and/or reduced auricular height.[20–22] Satyr ear is a form of lop ear, specifically with overfolding of the

TREATMENT TECHNIQUES

Many of the more common or subtle congenital auricular anomalies are best treated nonsurgically.[7] Molding can be a very successful alternative to surgical correction. When molding is placed for infants seen with deformities within the first week of life, success rates can be greater

---

Box 2
Classification of constricted ears

Tanzer Classification of Constricted Ears

- Group I: flattening or folding of the helix only
- Group II: abnormalities of the helix and scapha
  - Group IIA: moderate constriction, requiring no extra skin for repair
  - Group IIB: more severe, involving both antihelical crura, antihelical flattening, and/or hooding, requiring extra skin to expand the auricular margin
- Group III: auricle rolled into nearly tubular form

Daniali Classification of Constricted Ears

- Class I: shortened longitudinal axis, flattened superior crus, mild helical hooding, present scapha, mild prominence
- Class II: shortened longitudinal axis, absent superior crus, moderate helical hooding, shortened scapha, increased prominence
- Class III: severely shortened longitudinal axis, absent superior crus, severe helical hooding, obliterated scapha, severe prominence

than 90%.[31] Cartilage appears to be most pliable at birth, with high plasma concentrations of maternal estrogen, which decreases rapidly by 6 weeks of life to basal levels. Therefore, splinting therapies have been recommended for neonates with obvious deformities. Early molding may be used for a variety of auricular deformities, including prominent ear, cup ear, lop ear, Stahl ear, and constricted ears, especially Tanzer II. Traditionally, a hybrid of methods including individualized molding and taping was used. More recently, Byrd and colleagues[31] created the Ear-Well Infant Ear Correction System, a device standardizing the molding process while applying the principles in **Box 3**. This device has been used successfully in multiple studies and may decrease the molding time from 6 to 8 weeks in traditional methods to as little as 2 weeks.[19,31,32]

Surgical repair is typically recommended between the ages of 3 and 6 years old (the senior author's (APS) preference is between 5 and 6 years old) to minimize negative social impact.[33] Furthermore, surgical repair at younger ages allows the surgeon to rely more on cartilage-shaping techniques rather than cartilage-weakening techniques, as the auricular cartilage is more malleable when patients are younger. Goals of otoplasty are shown in **Box 4**.[34]

Cryptotia

The goals of cryptotia repair include creating a new auriculocephalic sulcus, correction of any deformed antihelical cartilage, and dissection of any abnormal auricular muscles, particularly the superior auricular muscle, auricular oblique muscle, and transverse auricular muscle.[21,35–38] Nearly all repairs consist of a posteriorly based flap, combined with a cartilage graft.

Posteriorly based flaps that expose the posterior aspect of the scapha are generally used. A Z-plasty technique may be used.[36] The central arm of the Z-plasty is drawn from the shortest line beginning from the hairline, across the temporoauricular sulcus, to the posterior scaphoid fossa

in a posterosuperior direction. The cranial lateral arm extends along the hairline beyond the cephaloauricular sulcus. The caudal lateral arm extends to the temporoauricular sulcus. Ideally, the angle between the central and the cranial lateral arm is greater than 60°, and the angle between the central and the caudal lateral arm is less than 45°. The larger cranial flap is later rotated to cover the posterior auricle, while the caudal flap is advanced cranially.

A modified trefoil flap may be used instead.[37] This method consists of 2 opposing flaps from the auricle and the scalp. The superior aspect of the helical rim is the base of the auricular trefoil flap and the apex of the opposing scalp trefoil flap. Each flap consists of 3 symmetric triangles, with the helical root and posterior cryptotic portion of the ear as the anterior and posterior borders, respectively. The apices of the triangles end in the hairline such that hair is not displaced into the new auriculocephalic sulcus. The scalp flap is widely undermined and advanced inferiorly to create the new sulcus.

Yet another method is the double V-Y advancement flap.[38] The first supra-auricular flap consists of the most anterior part of the buried ascending helix and the posterior auriculocephalic sulcus as the anterior and posterior limbs, respectively. The second retroauricular flap meets with the first flap on the posterior auricular surface (**Fig. 5**).

If the antihelical cartilage is deformed, a piece of conchal cartilage may be harvested for repair. It may be fixed to the superior portion of the cephaloauricular angle between the posterior antihelical cartilage and mastoid periosteum to enhance helical projection.[21] It may be applied as a strut graft internally if the antihelical cartilage is collapsed, or externally if the deformity is secondary to an irregular contour.[38]

Stahl Ear

Repairing the Stahl ear deformity requires excision of the third crus and formation of the missing

---

Box 3
Principles of auricular molding

- Continuation of the antihelical fold in the superior limb of the triangular fossa must be created with a stent resting along the retroauricular sulcus in direct alignment with the antihelix
- A curved anterior stent is also necessary along the helical rim to direct forces anteriorly in the scapha
- The helical rim must also be retracted to allow for expansion. If there is no helical rim development, then it must be created
- An anterior force also must be applied to flatten any conchal crus and correct the conchomastoid angle

Box 4
Goals of otoplasty

- Correct all protrusion in the upper one-third of the ear
- The helix of both ears should be able to be seen beyond the antihelix from the front
- The helix should be smooth and regular throughout
- The postauricular sulcus should not be significantly distorted or decreased
- The posterior measurement of the ear from the outer edge of the helix to the mastoid should be approximately 10 to 12 mm superiorly, 16 to 18 mm in the middle, and 20 to 22 mm inferiorly
- The position of the 2 ears should match within 3 mm at any given point

superior crus.[39–44] Any abnormal auricular muscles, particularly the often implicated transverse auricular muscle, should be identified and dissected.[16] The skin incision is typically made posteriorly along the desired site of the superior crus and antihelix. An anterior, scaphoid fossa incision also can be used to elevate an anterior flap. The cartilage is then exposed. The third crus may then be excised and positioned as a graft or rotated as a flap, after which the anterior flap is replaced (**Fig. 6**).[45,46] It alternatively may be scored, along with the surrounding posterior scapha and molded to produce the superior crus. If more cartilage is required, conchal cartilage may be harvested to create the superior crus. Mustarde

sutures from the posterior scaphoid fossa to the posterior conchal surface may be used to enhance the folding of the superior crus and antihelix.[44] Furnas sutures from the concha to the mastoid may be used for conchal setback.[43]

Cup Ear

The goals of cup ear repair include decreasing the conchoscaphal angle, producing a more prominent antihelical fold, and elongating the upper pole.[43,44,47–51] A posterior incision is often used to expose the posterior auricular cartilage and the posterior aspect of the helix. The auricular cartilage may then be incised from the lower pole

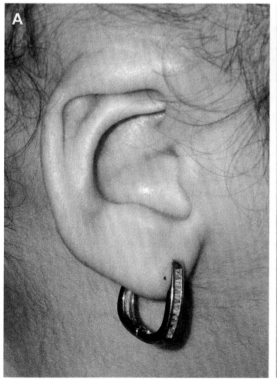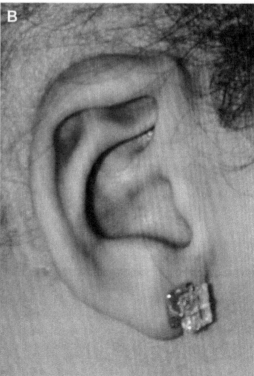

Fig. 5. Cryptotia. (*A*) Preoperative view. (*B*) Postoperative view.

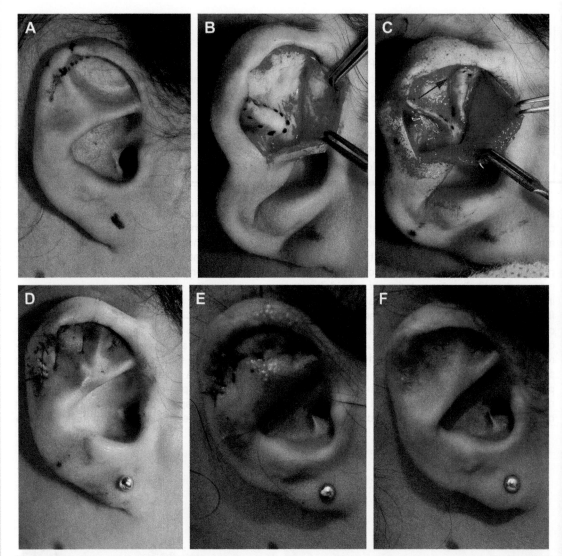

Fig. 6. Stahl deformity repair. (*A*) Preoperative marking shows position of anterior incision within the depth of the scaphoid fossa. (*B*) Anteriorly based flap elevated with perichondrium exposed cartilaginous upper third of the auricle. "Third crus" is outlined. (*C*) The third crus has been excised and grafted into the desired position of the superior crus (*arrow*) and will be sutured in place. Defect left at site of third crus shaved flush with surrounding cartilage. (*D*) Skin flap replaced and wound closed, mattress sutures placed in scaphoid fossa and fossa triangularis. Wound is dressed in a mineral oil–soaked cotton gauze and mastoid dressing. Earrings were placed at the time of surgery and made the focus of the procedure to distract the child. (*E*) Postoperative day 3. (*F*) Postoperative day 24.

of the antihelix to the anterior crus, parallel to the helical rim to reach the anterior surface. The skin may then be undermined off the anterior auricular cartilage, across the antihelix and into the concha. The perichondrium of the anterior auricular cartilage may then be scored, extending into the conchal cartilage if a deep concha needs correcting.[48] Excision of an ellipse of conchal cartilage may be necessary for deep conchal bowls.[47] This cartilage also may be used to repair a deformed helical rim or for reinforcement.

Trimming of the cauda helicis and excision of any elliptical or dumbbell-shaped segment of postauricular skin may be needed.

When the helical root and the scapha are both involved, a flap may need to be raised. A posteriorly based V-Y advancement flap may be used to advance the helical root.[49] The method is similar to that described previously for the double V-Y advancement flap (see Cryptotia section), but it is designed with 1 V, with its base along the helix to release the constricted ear (**Fig. 7**). Alternatively,

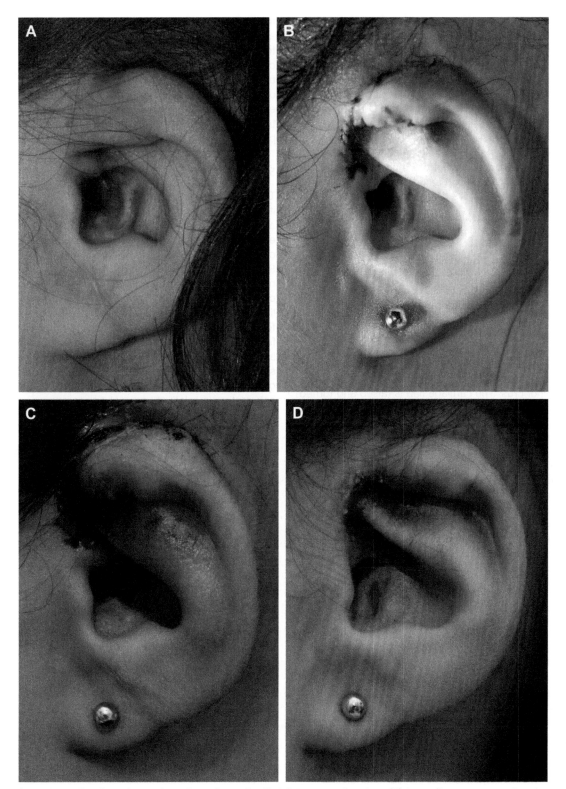

Fig. 7. Constricted ear (contralateral ear from **Fig. 6**). (*A*) Preoperative view. (*B*) Immediate postoperative view after V-Y rotation-advancement of helical root and anterior helical rim. (*C*) Postoperative day 3. (*D*) Postoperative day 24.

a Z-plasty advancement flap, as described previously (see Cryptotia section), may be used as yet another method.

These flaps may be combined with the use of various sutures to further shape the auricle. Mustarde sutures may be used if the antihelix is weak or absent, or if the cartilage is thin and compliant, to achieve the desired conchoscaphal angle.[44] Furnas sutures also may be used to correct a deep conchal bowl.[43] A mastoid stitch may be used to suture the upper neohelix to the mastoid fascia to maintain helical elevation and prevent recurrence.

Lop Ear

The primary goal of lop ear repair is to correct the deformed antihelix.[20–22] The most commonly used methods include various forms of cartilage shaping. The skin incision may be made on the lateral rim down to the perichondrium, raising the skin flap over the lateral scaphal surface toward the medial surface.[22] Any excess cartilage is then excised. The cartilage flap is then marked on the prominence of the antihelix, with its base at the inferior aspect of the inferior crus. An incision is then made at the location of the desired superior crus. The cartilage flap is raised and turned 180°, filling the defect and then sutured. This flap pushes the helix upward and increases the vertical height of the auricle.

Alternatively, a tumbling concha-cartilage flap may be used.[20] Either an anterior or posterior skin incision may be made but must include the entire vertical length of the concha in the flap. The conchal cartilage flap is then raised, tumbled backward, and passed through a tunnel under the postauricular skin. The tip of the cartilage flap is then fixed to the helix or scapha. The recoiling force of the cartilage will pull the anteriorly positioned helix or scapha back into the proper position.

Macrotia

Correcting macrotia involves reducing the helical rim, such that the upper third of the auricle contributes to approximately one-third of the final overall height.[29,52,53] An incision may be made in the retroauricular sulcus and just inside the helical rim on the lateral auricle for access.[52] A crescent-shaped segment of the scaphal cartilage may then be excised. A small segment of helical rim should also be excised to fit the reduced scapha. The helical rim may then be reapproximated primarily.

Alternatively, a double helical chondrocutaneous advancement flap may be used.[53,54] Two full-thickness skin and cartilage incisions should be made from the helical rim to the helical sulcus superior and inferiorly to produce 2 advancement flaps. The inferior helical flap may be extended as far as the upper lobule, and the superior flap to the helical root. The resulting double chondrocutaneous flaps are then reapproximated using a transient fixation suture to determine the amount of scaphal cartilage to be resected. A crescent of excess scapha is then excised, helical rims trimmed as necessary, and the incisions closed primarily.

SUMMARY

The gentle and intricate concavities and convexities of the auricle are instantly recognizable, and absence or malformation of any of these is easily recognized. Among the less common congenital auricular deformities are cryptotia, Stahl ear, constricted ear, and macrotia. Otoplasty to correct these anomalies must take into consideration the wide variety of these anomalies, even within these categorizations. Thus, the techniques used vary as widely as there are differences in these anomalies. Although patients and parents must understand that the reconstructed auricle will never exactly match the opposite side, surgery to repair these deformities can restore a relatively normal appearance and avoid the psychosocial and emotional issues associated with a facial deformity.

REFERENCES

1. Harris J, Kallen B, Robert E. The epidemiology of anotia and microtia. J Med Genet 1996;33(10): 809–13.
2. Jaffe BF. The incidence of ear diseases in the Navajo Indians. Laryngoscope 1969;79(12):2126–34.
3. Rubin LR, Bromberg BE, Walden RH, et al. An anatomic approach to the obtrusive ear. Plast Reconstr Surg Transpl Bull 1962;29:360–70.
4. Preuss S, Eriksson E. Prominent ears. In: Achauer BM, Eriksson E, Guyuron B, et al, editors. Plastic surgery: indications, operations and outcomes. St Louis (MO): Mosby; 2000. p. 1057–65.
5. Porter CJ, Tan ST. Congenital auricular anomalies: topographic anatomy, embryology, classification, and treatment strategies. Plast Reconstr Surg 2005;115(6):1701–12.
6. Yotsuyanagi T, Nihei Y, Shinmyo Y, et al. Stahl's ear caused by an abnormal intrinsic auricular muscle. Plast Reconstr Surg 1999;103(1):171–4.
7. Matsuo K, Hayashi R, Kiyono M, et al. Nonsurgical correction of congenital auricular deformities. Clin Plast Surg 1990;17(2):383–95.
8. Guyuron B, DeLuca L. Ear projection and the posterior auricular muscle insertion. Plast Reconstr Surg 1997;100(2):457–60.

9. Hirose T, Tomono T, Matsuo K, et al. Cryptotia: our classification and treatment. Br J Plast Surg 1985; 38(3):352–60.

10. Elsahy NI. An alternative technique for correction of cryptotia. Ann Plast Surg 1989;23(1):66–73.

11. Simon F, Celerier C, Garabedian EN, et al. Mastoid fascia kite flap for cryptotia correction. Int J Pediatr Otorhinolaryngol 2016;90:210–3.

12. Yotsuyanagi T, Yamauchi M, Yamashita K, et al. Abnormality of auricular muscles in congenital auricular deformities. Plast Reconstr Surg 2015;136(1): 78e–88e.

13. Matsuo K, Hirose T, Tomono T, et al. Nonsurgical correction of congenital auricular deformities in the early neonate: a preliminary report. Plast Reconstr Surg 1984;73(1):38–51.

14. Ferraro GA, Perrotta A, Rossano F, et al. Stahl syndrome in clinical practice. Aesthetic Plast Surg 2006;30(3):348–9 [discussion: 350].

15. Konaklioglu M, Ozmen OA, Unal OF. Stahl syndrome (Satiro's ear). Otolaryngol Head Neck Surg 2007; 137(4):674–5.

16. Gleizal A, Bachelet JT. Aetiology, pathogenesis, and specific management of Stahl's ear: role of the transverse muscle insertion. Br J Oral Maxillofac Surg 2013;51(8):e230–233.

17. Paik YS, Chang CW. Stahl ear deformity associated with Finlay-Marks syndrome. Ear Nose Throat J 2010;89(6):256–7.

18. Tanzer RC. The constricted (cup and lop) ear. Plast Reconstr Surg 1975;55(4):406–15.

19. Daniali LN, Rezzadeh K, Shell C, et al. Classification of newborn ear malformations and their treatment with the earwell infant ear correction system. Plast Reconstr Surg 2017;139(3):681–91.

20. Park C. The tumbling concha-cartilage flap for correction of lop ear. Plast Reconstr Surg 2000; 106(2):259–65.

21. Ho K, Boorer C, Khan U, et al. Innovative technique for correction of the congenital lop ear. J Plast Reconstr Aesthet Surg 2006;59(5):494–8.

22. Elsahy NI. Technique for correction of lop ear. Plast Reconstr Surg 1990;85(4):615–20.

23. Smith DW, Takashima H. Ear muscles and ear form. Birth Defects Orig Artic Ser 1980;16(4): 299–302.

24. Edwards MJ, McDonald D, Moore P, et al. Scalp-ear-nipple syndrome: additional manifestations. Am J Med Genet 1994;50(3):247–50.

25. Leung AK, Kong AY, Robson WL, et al. Dominantly-inherited lop ears. Am J Med Genet A 2007; 143A(19):2330–3.

26. O'Callaghan M, Young ID. The Townes-Brocks syndrome. J Med Genet 1990;27(7):457–61.

27. Rossmiller DR, Pasic TR. Hearing loss in Townes-Brocks syndrome. Otolaryngol Head Neck Surg 1994;111(3 Pt 1):175–80.

28. Farkas LG. Anthropometry of the normal and defective ear. Clin Plast Surg 1990;17(2):213–21.

29. Yuen A, Coombs CJ. Reduction otoplasty: correction of the large or asymmetric ear. Aesthetic Plast Surg 2006;30(6):675–8.

30. Gault DT, Grippaudo FR, Tyler M. Ear reduction. Br J Plast Surg 1995;48(1):30–4.

31. Byrd HS, Langevin CJ, Ghidoni LA. Ear molding in newborn infants with auricular deformities. Plast Reconstr Surg 2010;126(4):1191–200.

32. Doft MA, Goodkind AB, Diamond S, et al. The newborn butterfly project: a shortened treatment protocol for ear molding. Plast Reconstr Surg 2015;135(3):577e–83e.

33. Petersson RS, Friedman O. Current trends in otoplasty. Curr Opin Otolaryngol Head Neck Surg 2008;16(4):352–8.

34. McDowell AJ. Goals in otoplasty for protruding ears. Plast Reconstr Surg 1968;41(1):17–27.

35. Kubo I. Cryptotia and otoplasty. Jpn Otorhinolaryngology 1933;6:105–9.

36. Yotsuyanagi T, Yamashita K, Shinmyo Y, et al. A new operative method of correcting cryptotia using large Z-plasty. Br J Plast Surg 2001;54(1): 20–4.

37. Adams MT, Cushing S, Sie K. Cryptotia repair: a modern update to the trefoil flap. Arch Facial Plast Surg 2011;13(5):355–8.

38. Kim YS. Correction of cryptotia with upper auricular deformity: double V-Y advancement flap and cartilage strut graft techniques. Ann Plast Surg 2013; 71(4):361–4.

39. Kaplan HM, Hudson DA. A novel surgical method of repair for Stahl's ear: a case report and review of current treatment modalities. Plast Reconstr Surg 1999;103(2):566–9.

40. Kim SM, Kwon BY, Jun YJ, et al. Innovative method to correct Stahl ear that involves full thickness scoring incisions and an onlay graft of cymba conchal cartilage. Br J Oral Maxillofac Surg 2017; 55(1):81–3.

41. Liu L, Pan B, Lin L, et al. A new method to correct Stahl's ear. J Plast Reconstr Aesthet Surg 2011; 64(1):48–52.

42. Weinfeld AB. Stahl's ear correction: synergistic use of cartilage abrading, strategic Mustarde suture placement, and anterior anticonvexity suture. J Craniofac Surg 2012;23(3):901–5.

43. Furnas DW. Correction of prominent ears by concha-mastoid sutures. Plast Reconstr Surg 1968;42(3): 189–93.

44. Mustarde JC. The correction of prominent ears using simple mattress sutures. Br J Plast Surg 1963;16: 170–8.

45. Nakajima T, Yoshimura Y, Kami T. Surgical and conservative repair of Stahl's ear. Aesthetic Plast Surg 1984;8(2):101–7.

46. Gundeslioglu AO, Ince B. Stahl ear correction using the third crus cartilage flap. Facial Plast Surg 2013; 29(6):520–4.

47. Scharer SA, Farrior EH, Farrior RT. Retrospective analysis of the Farrior technique for otoplasty. Arch Facial Plast Surg 2007;9(3):167–73.

48. Chait L, Nicholson R. One size fits all: a surgical technique for the correction of all types of prominent ears. Plast Reconstr Surg 1999;104(1):190–5 [discussion: 196–7].

49. Elshahat A, Lashin R. Reconstruction of moderately constricted ears by combining V-Y advancement of helical root, conchal cartilage graft, and mastoid hitch. Eplasty 2016;16:e19.

50. Chongchet VA. Method of antihelix reconstruction. Br J Plast Surg 1963;16:268–72.

51. Horlock N, Grobbelaar AO, Gault DT. 5-year series of constricted (lop and cup) ear corrections: development of the mastoid hitch as an adjunctive technique. Plast Reconstr Surg 1998;102(7):2325–32 [discussion: 2333–5].

52. Sinno S, Chang JB, Thorne CH. Precision in otoplasty: combining reduction otoplasty with traditional otoplasty. Plast Reconstr Surg 2015;135(5): 1342–8.

53. Tezel E, Ozturk CN. Double helical rim advancement flaps with scaphal resection: selected cases over 10 years and review of the literature. Aesthetic Plast Surg 2011;35(4):545–52.

54. Antia NH, Buch VI. Chondrocutaneous advancement flap for the marginal defect of the ear. Plast Reconstr Surg 1967;39(5):472–7.

Autologous Rib Microtia Construction
Nagata Technique

Akira Yamada, MD, PhD

KEYWORDS

- Nagata technique • Microtia • Autogenous cartilage reconstruction • 6 types ear templates

KEY POINTS

- To achieve excellent outcomes of microtia reconstruction, all 3 keys, skin envelope, 3D framework, and proper location, must be perfect.
- Lobule split technique is the hallmark of the Nagata technique, which allows to expand skin surface area, and enables to create deeper conchal cavity.
- Six types of ear framework templates were developed by the author, based on the curve analysis of normal auricles, and these templates have been used for microtia patients in all ethnic groups.
- To master 3D cartilage framework creation, surgeons must practice intensely before starting clinical cases. For that purpose, the author's personal training method is described.

INTRODUCTION

I became Satoru Nagata's disciple in 1997, and spent 3.5 years with him.

We operated together for approximately 400 cases of autogenous rib microtia construction. Before Nagata developed his technique, autogenous rib microtia construction was a 4-stage to 6-stage procedure, and Nagata transformed it to a 2-stage total ear reconstruction. The Nagata technique is technically demanding, but the author loves this technique because of the aesthetically pleasing and sustainable outcomes. Since his landmark article in 1993, there are substantial changes in his techniques. The author modified the Nagata technique in terms of framework templates, otherwise the author tries to use Nagata's latest techniques. To achieve satisfactory, long-standing outcomes, surgeons must execute 3 key components perfectly: well-vascularized supple skin envelope, precise 3-dimensional (3D) framework, and anatomically proper ear location.

In this article, the author explains how the analysis and planning of the Nagata technique is performed to achieve aesthetically pleasing autogenous rib microtia construction.

EAR LOCATION

If you carefully observe the articles/textbook chapters written by the "Giants" of ear reconstruction, such as Tanzer,[1,2] Brent,[3] and Nagata,[4–6] you may notice one thing in common. They are very careful to place a new auricle in the aesthetically pleasing location. This is often ignored by less experienced surgeons. Planning to place the new ear in the aesthetically pleasing location is actually the key to achieve successful ear reconstruction. Anatomically if you project the auricle on the facial skeleton, the auricle sits on the temporal bone, far back from the facial triangle. The auricle is located just outside of the face mask (**Fig. 1**). The auricle is at least 1 ear-length behind the lateral canthus[7,8] (**Fig. 2**). The

Disclosure Statement: Dr A. Yamada is a nonpaid consultant for KLS Martin, which is making microtia surgical instruments.
World Craniofacial Foundation, 7777 Forest Lane Suite C-616, Dallas, TX 75230, USA
E-mail address: akira.yamada@worldcf.org

Facial Plast Surg Clin N Am 26 (2018) 41–55
https://doi.org/10.1016/j.fsc.2017.09.006
1064-7406/18/© 2017 Elsevier Inc. All rights reserved.

Location of the Auricle

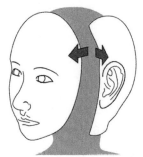

• Auricle is not located in the face mask

Fig. 1. Auricle is located just outside of face mask. (*Courtesy of* Toshinobu Harada, PhD, Wakayama-City, Japan.)

top of the auricle is usually at the level of the eyebrow, and the bottom of the auricle is at the level of the alar base. The auricle is tilted posteriorly 10 to 15°(s). The common mistake is to place the auricle upright, or even tilted forward, in an effort to avoid postero-lateral hairline, using preauricular skin as a part of the new auricle.

DIMENSION OF EAR SHAPE

The width of the well-proportioned ear is 50% to 55% of the length (**Fig. 3**). The Frankfurt horizontal

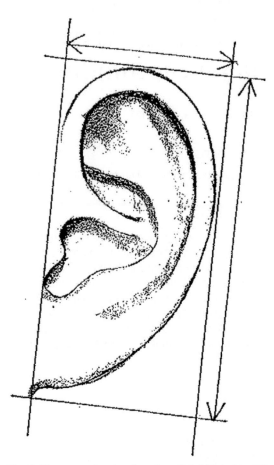

Fig. 3. The normal ratio of ear-length/width is 1 to 0.5 to 0.55. (*Modified from* Tolleth H. Artistic anatomy, dimensions, and proportions of the external ear. Clinics in Plastic Surgery 1978;5(3)337; with permission.)

line is located at the upper edge of tragus, and divides the auricle into upper and lower halves (see **Fig. 2**). The width of the helix is 10% of its length. The tragus must be located in the second vertical quartile from the lower end. The axis measurement is difficult to define, but 15 to 20° appears to be a satisfactory angle.[9] Some indicate the axis to be parallel to the bridge of the nose, but it is not always true for both adults and children.

EAR SHAPE ANALYSIS

Normal auricle shape is made of multiple smooth curves that include the spiral curve of the helix (**Fig. 4**). Therefore, one of the most important aspects of total auricular construction is how we create natural-looking curves in the new auricle.

Nagata uses a single ideal ear template he developed for all cases. The author used Nagata ear templates for the first 10 years, and I observed

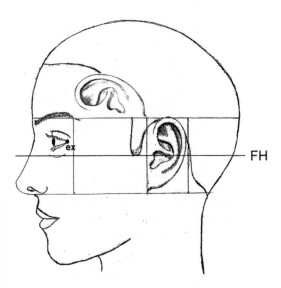

Fig. 2. The proper location of the auricle; the auricle is at least 1 ear-length behind the lateral canthus. (*Modified from* Tolleth H. Artistic anatomy, dimensions, and proportions of the external ear. Clinics in Plastic Surgery 1978;5(3)337; with permission.)

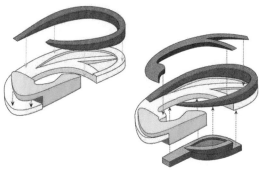

Fig. 4. The architecture of the ear framework; helix (*red*) is a spiral structure, connecting the first floor (*bottom* of the base frame) to the second floor (on *top* of the base frame). (*Courtesy of* Toshinobu Harada, PhD, Wakayama-City, Japan.)

in my own outcomes that there were slight differences of ear shape despite using the same ear template. Then the author began to explore what is making of ear shape difference for each individual.

Harada and colleagues[10] defined there are 2 key curves in the normal auricle: helix-lobule curve and concha outline curve. A Japanese study shows that there are 3 major types of helix-lobule curve (**Fig. 5**), and 2 major types of concha outline curves (**Fig. 6**). Based on these 2 key curves of the auricle, Harada and colleagues[10] classified the normal auricle shape into 6 types (**Fig. 7**).

Based on this classification, 6 types of normal ear templates are created for auricular construction, and since 2009 the author has used these clinical cases. The author applied 6 types of ear templates for autogenous rib microtia reconstruction in 25 academic universities around the globe. Based on these experiences with microtia patients of varying ethnic backgrounds, I believe that 6 types of ear templates can be applied to microtia patients of all ethnic backgrounds.

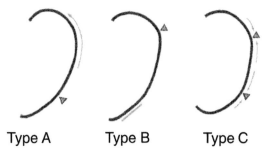

Type A   Type B   Type C

Fig. 5. The classification of helix-lobule curve: there are 3 major types in the healthy population; Type A, Type B, and Type C. *Arrowhead* indicates inflection point (meaning the abrupt change of the curve ratio).

PREOPERATIVE PLANNING

The purpose of preoperative planning is to assess the types of deformities of the patient, and the surgical strategy tailored to the individual deformities. The accurate identification of the auricular rectangle and its relation to the vestige will determine the difficulty of the case. Proper preoperative planning is crucial to avoid misguided surgical strategy.

Timing of Surgery

The Brent method requires less cartilage, thus 6 to 7 years old may be the timing for surgery. The Nagata method, on the other hand, requires a larger amount of 6 to 9 ipsilateral costal cartilage stock, with the following recommended criteria of surgery:

1. 10 years of age
2. Chest circumference of 60 cm at the lowest sternum level (xiphoid)

Check the Skin Quality

The skin quality around the ear area greatly influences the outcome. For example, scar tissue will interfere with the natural expansion of skin and can cause poor definition of ear shape. In case of a larger area of scar tissues near the ear site, you may need to consider the use of fascia flap to augment the supple skin envelope. Even without scar tissue, skin elasticity varies individually and this factor will influence the definition of the ear. Hence, the author always checks the skin elasticity at both the ear site and rib cartilage donor site, trying to predict the skin elasticity during surgery as a mental preparation for surgery; if the patient has relatively tight skin, the author considers creating a 1-mm lower-profile 3D framework, to avoid strain to the skin envelope.

Identify Auricular Rectangle

Even in a symmetric face, some surgeons do not pay attention to the precise location of the new auricle. The location of the auricle, however, is as important as the ear shape itself to achieve an aesthetically pleasing outcome. "Auricular rectangle" is the term the author coined to clarify the importance of identifying the proper location of the new ear (**Fig. 8**). It helps to decide if the vestige is located in a surgically usable location at the same timing of 3D frame implantation. If the vestige is located outside of the auricular rectangle, especially located more than 1.0 to 1.5 cm away from the rectangle, separate surgery to

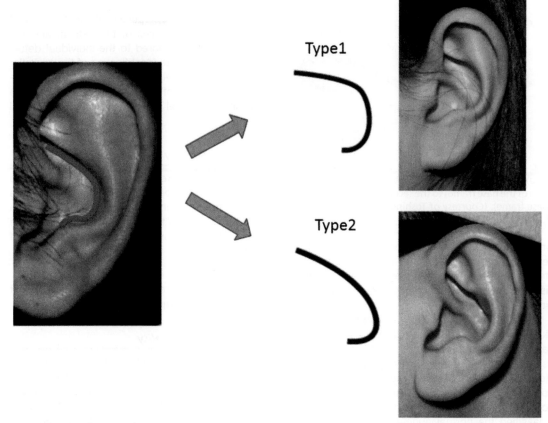

Fig. 6. The classification of concha outline; there are 2 major types of concha outline in the healthy population; type 1 and type 2.

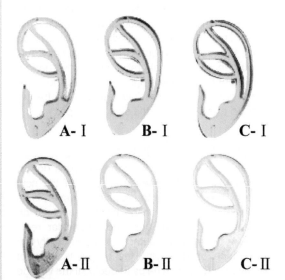

Fig. 7. Six types of normal ear template (3 × 2 = 6) are developed to express the nuance of normal auricular curves. There are three major types (Type A,B,C) of helix-lobule curve, and two major curves of concha outline (Type 1and 2) in healthy population.

transpose the vestige before framework implantation may be necessary.

Avoid Dissecting "Preauricular Trapezoid"

If you observe the normal anatomy in front of the auricle, you will see non–hair-bearing skin shaped like a trapezoid (**Fig. 9**). I coined the term "preauricular trapezoid," where skin perforators that give blood supplies to the auricle exist. We are still investigating which specific perforators would be dominant, and critical for the auricular skin. The author recommends not violating this area to secure the blood supplies to the new ear. Avoiding preauricular trapezoid area dissection also helps to prevent anterior inclination of the new ear, which is a common mistake in auricular construct.

Managing Hairline

Nobody wants hairs growing on the ear, hence surgeons tend to avoid the hairline and place the new ear in too upright a position, consuming non–hair-bearing preauricular skin. Anthropometric study shows that 10 to 15° posterior

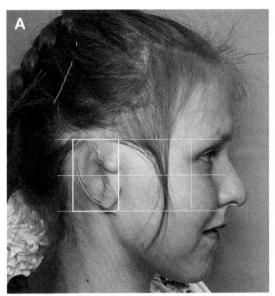
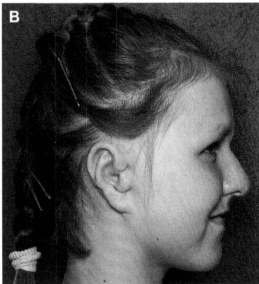

Fig. 8. (*A*) The first step of microtia reconstruction is to identify the "auricular rectangle" in which the new auricle will be constructed. (*B*) The clinical outcome after the first stage of autogenous rib cartilage ear reconstruction.

inclination is natural, and aesthetically pleasing. Too upright an ear is not aesthetically attractive.[8] If the ear will involve hairs in more than 15% of the framework area, augmenting the skin envelope with a fascia flap should be considered. Fewer than 15% of hairs may be removed at the second-stage surgery by using intraoperative epilation techniques. I do not recommend to

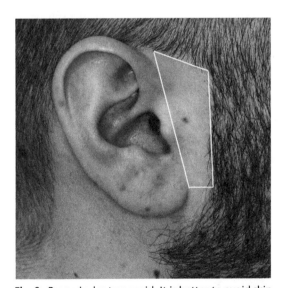

Fig. 9. Preauricular trapezoid. It is better to avoid skin flap dissection in this area for 2 reasons: perforator vessels to give blood supply to the auricle comes from this area, if you dissect this area, framework tends to be located too upright.

placing the 3D frame under thick hairs more than 15% of total ear height for 2 reasons: (1) the presence of thick hairs means that skin flap dissection at the time of 3D frame implantation was too thick to create the helical shape, and (2) laser hair epilation after 3D frame implantation may cause heat damage to the cartilage framework, because the hair follicles are almost touching the cartilage framework. It is important to note that laser hair epilation works best for black hairs, and less effectively against blond hairs. Even with black hairs, it may take more than 10 sessions to completely remove hairs permanently.

Ear-Positioning Template

The ear-positioning template (EPT) was developed by the author during the fellowship with Nagata in 1997. The role of EPT is to identify the optimal location to place the new auricle. EPT is made of overhead projector (OHP) film on which anatomic references are printed; ear template, Frankfurt horizontal line, and 2 parallel lines to it at superior and inferior margins of the template. EPT is transparent; therefore, the surgeon can draw the normal anatomy, reference landmarks of the normal side. Then EPT is reflected to the other side, and used to draw markings on the microtia side after intubation (**Fig. 10**).

Dystopic Vestige

Dystopic vestige (vestige lobule is located far below the alar base level, and also anteriorly

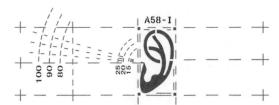

Fig. 10. EPT. EPT helps to identify the proper location of the new auricle.

dislocated) is commonly associated with hemifacial microsomia. Dystopic vestige is also frequently associated with low hair line. This combination is the common cause of dislocation of the new auricle. Surgeons tend to place the 3D framework in non–hair-bearing skin, thus the location of the ear becomes far below the normal level. Once the framework is placed in a wrong place, moving the implanted framework viable is extremely difficult. Therefore, the author strongly recommends that surgeons should carefully identify the proper location of the new auricle first, then surgical strategy should follow based on the location of the new ear, and its relationship with the surrounding anatomy. Transposing dystopia vestige cephalad may be the first-stage procedure, before 3D frame implantation.

Special Consideration for Secondary Construction

When you see patients presented with unsatisfactory outcomes, the author recommends checking the availability of the facial flap, especially temporoparietal fascia flap, and occipital fascia flap with Doppler ultrasound. The course of the artery use be traced long, up to the parietal area.

SURGICAL TECHNIQUES
First Stage

Preoperative marking after intubation, before preparation

It is critical to identify the "auricular rectangle" where the new ear is going to be built. Once you identify the auricular rectangle, you then can design the proper skin incision design. Again, if the vestige is too far away from the auricular rectangle, you will not be able to use the vestige simultaneously at the same time of 3D frame implantation.

The surgeon should know this before going into the operating room.

The author prefers to mark everything right after intubation, before preparation. Once the patient is prepped, it will be extremely difficult to spend time for marking in detail, because everybody is in a

hurry. The author routinely uses EPT to draw useful landmark information from the opposite normal site in unilateral microtia case (**Fig. 11**).

Ear template

Tracing a normal ear as an ear template is still a popular method (Tanzer/Brent) as a guide for making ear framework. I do not use the normal side as a template of ear shape for 3 reasons: (1) tracing the normal ear shape tends to be 1 to 2 mm larger than the cartilage framework, (2) template traced from the normal side tends to be too wide, and is likely to cause skin deficiency, and result in poor definition of the auricle, (3) capturing the characteristics of the normal side, and drawing an accurate curve from tracing is not an easy task, unless the surgeon is a professional artist. Therefore, I use 6 types of templates that we developed, based on the curve analysis of the auricle (see **Fig. 7**).

Lobule split technique

The lobule split techniques is a critical skin envelope preparation in the Nagata technique. Splitting the lobule allows us to place skin flaps in the concha cavity at the same time with 3D framework implantation. The lobule techniques have made departure of the Nagata method from previous methods (Tanzer, Brent) in terms of creation of a deep concha cavity. If the patient has enough volume of vestige lobule, it is possible to create a deep conchal cavity at the first stage of surgery. Secondary composite graft to create concha cavity (Brent) is no longer necessary. The author does not inject local anesthesia, because uneven injection could make splitting the lobule more difficult, and also makes it difficult to check the status of the vascular supply of the skin flap. The lobule flap technique is demanding, requires focus, and delicate soft tissue skills. It is best done first thing in the morning with fresh hands, instead of after

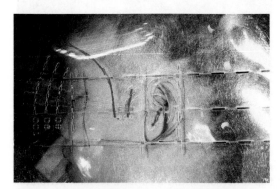

Fig. 11. Anatomic landmarks of the normal side are marked on EPT, and used to confirm the proper location of the new auricle.

harvesting rib cartilage. To prevent skin necrosis, the split must be done right in the middle to divide it evenly. Nagata recommends using a #15 scalpel for splitting the lobule. Holding the vestige softly between thumb and index finger with the sharp edge facing up, the lobule is split with multiple small stabbing motions. This is a blind maneuver; therefore, you must check the location of the tip of the blade from time to time to split in half. The vestige skin tends become thinner at the bottom, therefore very careful split is recommended, especially when getting closer to the base of the vestige (**Fig. 12**). The split of the lobule can stop when you see the fascia level. You will also see the vestige cartilage at this stage, and the next step would be to remove vestige cartilage; all of vestige needs to be removed for the lobule-type microtia, and the concha portion will be preserved for concha-type microtia.

Design of anterior lobule flap
The anterior lobule flap is designed to cover the anterior aspect of the lobule portion of 3D framework. This is made by splitting the vestige lobule. The width of skin pedicle should be wider than 9 mm according to Nagata to maintain sufficient vascularity.

Design of posterior flap
Nagata described the posterior skin flap as a W-shaped flap. The shape of the flap can be W or U shape, depend on the location and orientation of the vestige lobule (**Fig. 13**). Again, identification of the auricular rectangle will determine the proper

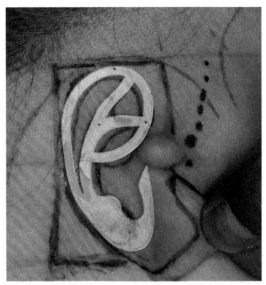

Fig. 13. Preoperative marking of the posterior skin flap; because of the vestige location, the design of the flap is not W-shaped, but U-shaped.

skin flap design. For concha-type microtia with abundant concha skin surface, you can use either a W-shaped flap or V-shaped flap. The anterior portion of posterior flap is attached to the subcutaneous pedicle to secure the vascular supply. This attachment also helps to keep the skin flap stuck to the 3D framework, preventing shallow concha depth. Deep concha is aesthetically important because it creates the shadow. Shadow at the concha makes the new ear more natural.

Avoid skin dissection in the "preauricular trapezoid"
Recent development of perforator flap revealed that there are numerous perforators to give blood supply to the normal auricle, located in front of the auricle. It is, however, still unknown whether there is any dominant perforators to supply the auricle. Therefore, I try not to violate the "preauricular trapezoid" (see **Fig. 8**) to preserve as much blood supply as possible. At the time of ear elevation, we must cut the blood supply from the posterior aspect; therefore, it makes sense to preserve the blood supply from the anterior aspect. Avoiding the "preauricular trapezoid" also helps to prevent anterior inclination of the auricle, which is considered not attractive.

Skin pocket dissection
It is important to note that skin dissection should be in 3 dimensions (upper, posterior, lower), and should avoid anterior dimension.

The skin pocket dissection must be done in uniform thickness, approximately 2-mm thick. The

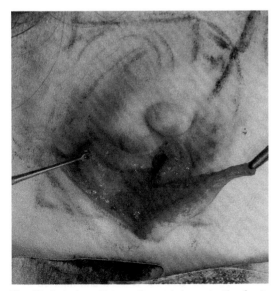

Fig. 12. Lobule split is performed down to the fascia level.

author uses small blunt straight scissors to facilitate this dissection. I do not recommend using curved scissors for non–hair-bearing skin pocket dissection, because it may create uneven skin flap thickness. Uneven thickness of skin flap may be the cause of skin necrosis. The junction between non–hair-bearing and hair-bearing skin needs complete freeing to avoid tension to the 3D framework. Incomplete dissection will cause bandlike tension in this area that may cause pressure to the 3D framework, which can lead to resorption/deformities. The author usually dissects 1 cm beyond the hairline to release the tension for the 3D framework.

The amount of subcutaneous pedicle
According to the original diagram illustrated by Nagata himself in 1993, the location of the subcutaneous pedicle is depicted as a "pinpoint." People misunderstood it as if the subcutaneous pedicle is small: that does not help augmenting the vascular supply. Do not create a subcutaneous pedicle pinpoint from the beginning, rather keep it reasonable in size and narrow it later as needed when placing the 3D framework in position. After the lobule is split, the next step for skin preparation is to do skin pocket dissection laterally. In this process, the surgeon will see the large amount of soft tissue attachment at the posterior skin flap. The author does not recommend making a subcutaneous pedicle too small (**Fig. 14**). The surgeon will need to create a space posterior to the transposed posterior flap. The author recommends lateral skin pocket dissection without making the pedicle too thin; you can then trim the size of the pedicle until the 3D frame can be inserted around the subcutaneous pedicle.

Harvesting rib cartilage
The author usually harvests ipsilateral sixth to ninth rib cartilage without perichondrium. Harvesting rib cartilage without perichondrium is a much safer technique than harvesting with perichondrium, because of one more layer of protection. Also, it is more likely to obtain the regeneration of cartilage/bone matrix, if you leave the perichondrium 100% to the donor site.[11] On the other hand, if you remove perichondrium together with the rib cartilage, the child may suffer from significant depressive chest deformities with less protection of the chest cage. The Nagata technique uses the leftover small pieces of cartilage; if relatively large pieces are left, they could be banked for the second-stage elevation, if the pieces are small, cartilage is diced into tiny pieces, and placed inside the sutured perichondrial pocket. This filling

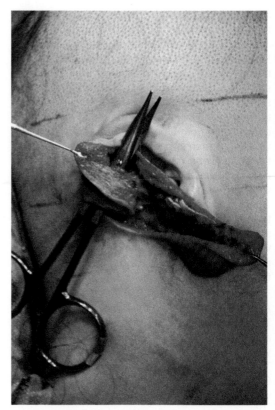

Fig. 14. Subcutaneous pedicle of the posterior flap is shown; note that the pedicle is not pinpoint, and has relatively large width.

of cartilage helps to bolster the regeneration of the cartilage (**Fig. 15**).

Balance between the amount of skin envelope and the height of 3D framework
During surgery, the surgeon should keep thinking about the balance between available skin envelope and the skin surface area required to cover the 3D framework. This balance is necessary to achieve clear definition of the auricle. If the vestige

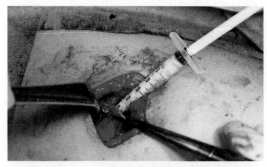

Fig. 15. Leftover cartilage is diced and injected into the space underneath the perichondrium to boost cartilage regeneration.

lobule is small, higher 3D framework may not work. If the patient has tight skin in quality, the 3D framework may need to lower 1 mm or so to avoid the skin circulation compromise.

Three-dimensional framework construct

The biggest difference between the 2D framework and the 3D framework is a "spiral stairs" (= helix) connecting the first layer (bottom of the base frame), to the second layer (helix) (**Fig. 16**). The author creates a smooth helix with 1 eighth full-length rib cartilage, instead of multiple pieces together. There are group of surgeons who do not connect the helix to the base frame, claiming that crus helicis should not be too obvious to show. However, the author strongly recommends connecting the helix to the bottom of the base frame, because this connection makes the framework far more stable; additionally, the complete spiral shape makes the framework more 3-dimensional. It is my observation that collapsed frameworks, when removed at the time of secondary ear construction, almost always did not connect the helix to the base frame. The antihelix is highest in the middle, and slowly slopes down toward the helix. Superior crus and inferior crus are going down the slope toward the lowest portion of the base frame. It is very important to secure enough space between the upper helix and superior and inferior crura, otherwise there will not be enough space to accommodate the skin envelope, and thus creating the unfavorable impression of continuity between 2 crura and helix. The total height of the 3D framework is 9.5 to 10.0 mm for primary cases, and maybe 1.0 to 2.0 mm higher for secondary cases. Rounding the posterior corner is important to avoid a "square-looking auricle," observed from behind. The latest Nagata framework includes 2 additional small pieces to make concha cymba, and concha cavum deeper. These 2 small pieces also help to stabilize the framework.

Fixation materials for 3D framework

When 2 cartilage pieces are connected by sutures or wires, it is my observation that these 2 pieces are less likely to fuse together like bone; instead, the connection between the 2 pieces of cartilage is mostly a fibrous connection. Therefore, the author recommends using fine wires to create 3D framework architecture, instead of Nylon sutures as a rigid fixation to obtain long-term stability. I suspect that a main reason of ear framework collapse in the long-term originates from less rigid fixation of the framework with Nylon sutures as compared with wire fixation.

Temporary suction to adapt the skin envelope

Skin trimming Skin trimming is the last procedure to come, at the time of maximum fatigue. This procedure needs patience and focus, and will determine the immediate success of the long-hour procedures. Temporary suction helps to determine the precise location, and the amount of skin to be trimmed. Nagata recommends trimming the skin to create traverse closure of the skin in the end. Temporary suction will be removed after the bolster sutures are in place.

Bolster sutures

A misconception about bolster sutures is that the bolster sutures are used to create the shape by giving pressure to the skin envelope. Before placing bolster sutures, the ear shape must be present there. The bolster sutures only help to maintain the shape. The real purposes of bolster sutures are (1) preventing hematoma formation, and (2) to form an adhesion between the skin flap and cartilage as seen with temporal suction. We should already have a clear definition of ear, before placing bolster sutures (**Fig. 17**). Sutures should be tied very gently to avoid any strain to the skin flaps. Never make the suture tie too tight. Wider grasp of skin width with large ark diameter needle is a safer technique to prevent skin vascular compromise.

Postoperative care Close follow-up is mandatory to avoid disastrous complications. The author checks the skin flap color almost every day for the first week postoperatively. The skin behind the bolster suture must be checked to avoid a pressure sore. Even the mildest tie of the bolster sutures, in 48 to 72 hours postoperative, at the time of maximum swelling, sutures may become tight. The author prepares 2 sterile forceps, a bright flashlight, ointment, and fluffy gauze for dressing change. Glasscock ear dressing is a

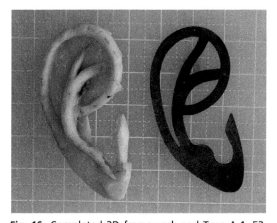

Fig. 16. Completed 3D framework and Type A-1, 52-mm template.

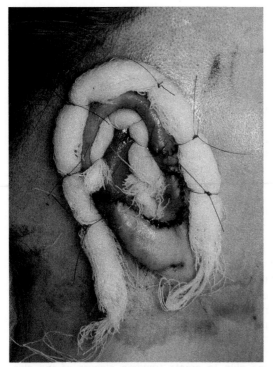

Fig. 17. The view of bolster sutures; it is vital to tie very gently.

convenient material both for protection and dressing change in a cool environment. In a hot and moist environment, however, Glasscock dressing may accumulate heat and moisture inside, and

may cause the skin color changes (red), and the red skin color may be confused with inflammation/infection. I make a larger hole in the Glasscock dome to release the heat and vapor, if needed.

The author instructs the patient/parents to keep the wound dry for 2 weeks. Shower below the neck will be ok after 1 week.

Second Stage

Second stage is the surgery to elevate the auricle from the head. Conventional "division" of the auricle from the head is to place skin grafting to the back of the auricle and the mastoid skin defect, and there is no anatomic skeletal support for elevation.

Because of lack of skeletal support, the ear is not elevated, and tends to contact with mastoid skin. As a result, this narrow space sometimes becomes difficult for the patient to clean. If you use groin skin as a source of skin graft, after puberty, grafted skin may grow curled pubic hairs.

The second stage of the Nagata technique is a more complex procedure than conventional division of the ear from the head: separate the auricle from the mastoid, harvest rib cartilage, create a wedge-shaped cartilage block and place it underneath the auricle, harvest a temporoparietal fascia (TPF) flap, transfer the TPF to cover the entire posterior aspect of the auricle, and finally graft split scalp skin on the fascia flap (**Fig. 18**). Split scalp

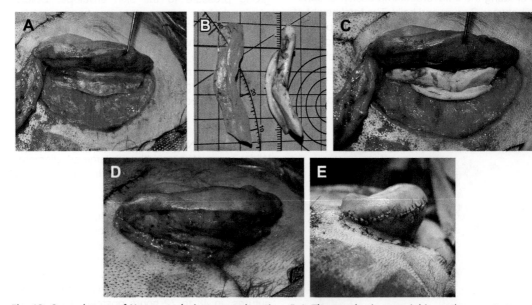

Fig. 18. Second stage of Nagata technique; ear elevation. R-1: Thermoelastic material is used to create template for cartilage grafting, with preoperative measurement of normal ear distance from head. R-2: cartilage graft for elevation is created according to the template. R-3: The cartilage is placed underneath the ear framework for elevation. R-4: TPF flap covers entire posterior aspect of the auricle. R-5: The view from the above showing the ear elevation, after split-thickness scalp is grafted over fascia flap.

skin has a better color match with skin of the anterior auricle than groin skin.

Secondary Ear Reconstruction

Secondary ear reconstruction is more challenging than primary reconstruction.[12] In most secondary cases, all 3 key components (skin envelope, framework, and ear location) are way off from the normal anatomy. Partial correction usually does not work well to improve the shape. Thus, a total redo may be the best option for many cases. New large skin envelope, and new 3D framework are necessary to create new auricle. If bilateral rib cartilages (6–9) are already consumed, although such a situation would be rare, surgeons

may need to use synthetic materials for 3D ear framework.

A case of secondary rib cartilage microtia construction

A 13-year-old girl, was operated on 3 times in another institution (**Fig. 19**). The reconstructed ear has thick hairs in the upper portion. The child and parents were unhappy about the construction and came to see the author. The presence of superficial temporal artery (STA) is confirmed at the outpatient clinic with Doppler ultrasound. Total ear reconstruction is planned. Surgical marking is simulated using a preoperative photo. After intubation, the patient was placed in a mild semilateral position, keeping the neck in a neutral

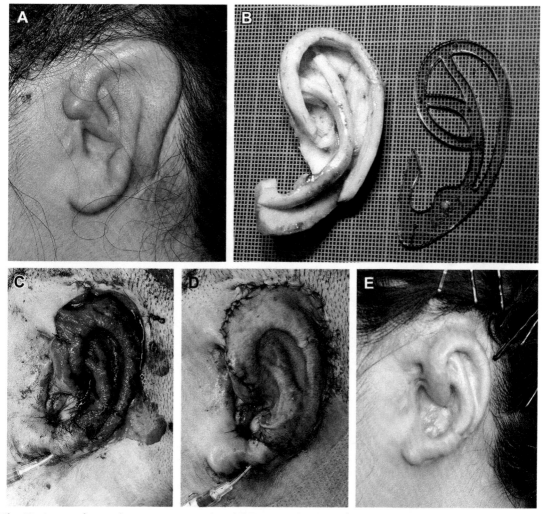

Fig. 19. A case of secondary ear reconstruction. (*A*) Preoperative view after tissue expansion method. (*B*) Created 3D framework and Type A-1 54-mm template. (*C*) Upper two-thirds of 3D framework is covered with temporoparietal fascia flap, and the lower one-third is covered with local skin flap. (*D*) Split-thickens scalp is placed over fascia coverage. (*E*) The view 1 year after the secondary construction.

position to prevent C1 C2 subluxation. Anatomic references are copied from the normal side drawn onto the EPT. With the help of EPT, preoperative markings are made, before the preparation. Two teams worked simultaneously; one team was working on the ear site, and the other team started to harvest the left rib cartilage. Scar tissues were removed as much as possible. The lobule was split into 2 flaps: anterior flap and posterior flap. The anterior lobule was brought cephalad into correct position, and the posterior flap was transpositioned up to the concha cavity. Attention was then turned to TPF flap, zig-zag incision was made, down to the hair bulb level. Skin flap was reflected just above the fascia layer, with careful sharp dissection with a #15 scalpel. STA was traced all the way to the parietal area, approximately 10 cm from the top of the auricle.

Wide dissection was made to allow visual confirmation of both artery and vein: a 6-7 × 10 cm TPF (temporoparietal fascia flap) was made. The 3D framework was created from 6 to 9 ipsilateral rib cartilage pieces. After copious irrigation with saline, perichondrium was closed halfway, diced leftover rib cartilage was placed into the space inside the perichondrium. Then perichondrial closure was completed. The wound closure was performed in layers. With help from EPT, the 3D frame was placed in proper anatomic location. The lower one-third of the frame was covered with the local skin flap. The upper two-thirds of the frame was covered with TPF, with temporal suction in place to adapt the TPF to the 3D framework; 5-0 Vicryl was used to seal the 3D frame with fascia flap, so as to adapt the fascia flap accurately. The temporal skin wound was closed in

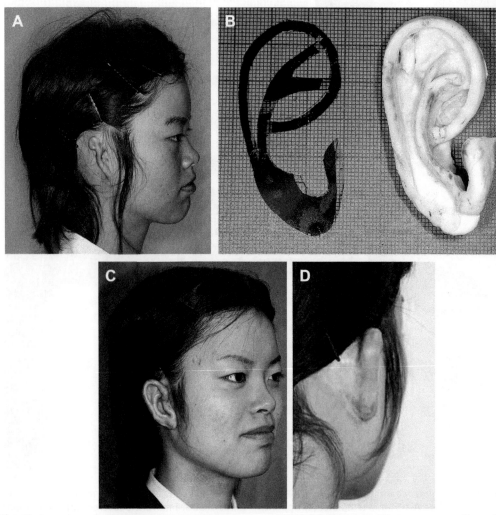

Fig. 20. Long-term follow-up of lobule-type microtia. (A) Preoperative view. (B) Autogenous rib cartilage 3D framework. (C) Eight years after surgery; oblique view. (D) Eight years after surgery; posterior view.

layers, after placing the suction drain. Split-thickness scalp skin, 12 to 13/1000-inch thickness, was harvested from the scalp, and was grafted on the fascia.

Meticulous skin closure was performed to stabilize the contour of the grafting. Finally, bolster sutures were placed carefully, avoiding puncturing the vessels. Temporary suction was removed, and the wound was completely closed. Reston dressing was placed around the wound for protection. Fluffy gauze was gently placed on the auricle.

LONG-TERM OUTCOMES

The author's personal cases show that Nagata techniques can produce sustainable outcomes in the long-term with minimum complications (**Fig. 20**).

COMPLICATIONS
Skin Flap Necrosis

During the first postoperative 10 days, the concern for surgeons is skin flap necrosis. Skin necrosis needs immediate attention, because it could lead to deeper cartilage infection and resorption of the framework. Immediate local skin flap or local fascia flap coverage will minimize the damage.

Infection

Infection is not a common complication in autogenous rib microtia construction. Vigorous irrigation and systemic antibiotics are necessary measures to save the cartilage framework.

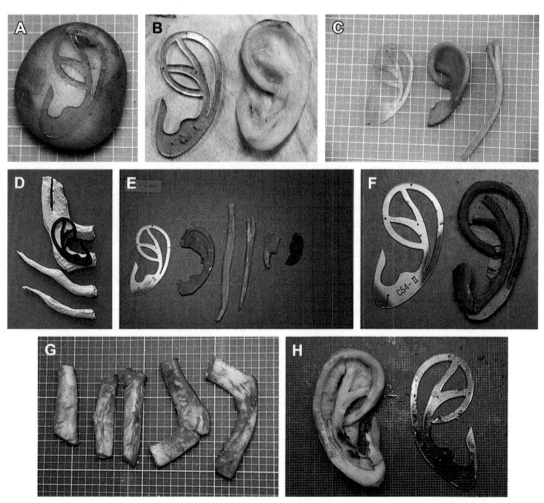

Fig. 21. Four-step training method of 3D frame carving. (*A*) The first step is carving practice using potato. (*B*) Completed potato framework and Type C 2, 54-mm template. (*C*) Step 2 training uses carrot to practice assembly of 5 parts of framework. (*D*) Step 3 is to simulate transforming rib cartilage shape into 3D ear framework, using precise copy of rib cartilage. (*E*) Five parts of 3D framework are shown: base framework, helix, antihelix, triages, and concha. (*F*) Completed 3D framework model, and Type C 2, 54-mm template. (*G*) Cartilage removed from the patient of pectus excavatum. (*H*) Completed 3D framework made from pectus excavatum cartilage.

Cartilage Resorption

Three-dimensional framework resorption and deformities are the consequences after ischemia or infection. A tight skin envelope, especially at the hairline border, could be the cause of helix resorption. This can be avoided by careful skin pocket dissection around the hair line. There is a kind of tight fibrous band along the hair line margin that needs to be released.

Wire Extrusion

The author uses 38-G wires, and they may extrude; 38-G wires are less likely to extrude than larger wires such as 34 G. Extruded wires can be removed at the outpatient clinic easily. It is important to educate patient/family to come to the clinic for wire removal as soon as extrusion is noticed. In rare circumstances, if wires are exposed for a prolonged period, it may cause mild resorption of cartilage around the wire.

SIMULATION TRAINING

Because the primary surgery is the key to achieve optimal outcome, surgeons must obtain more than enough training to achieve this goal; mastering basic reconstructive skills, such as delicate flap dissection, skin grafting, and delicate wound closures, are minimum requirements. In addition, surgeons must master precise carving/construction techniques for 3D ear framework. Importance of aesthetic judgment for proper ear location is often underestimated. Visiting expert surgeon for a short period of time is usually not enough to achieve this goal.

Education/training to become an "ear maker" was not well developed until recently. Simulation surgery has been reported by a few, aiming to minimize the experimental or practicing surgeries by inexperienced surgeons.

The author developed a 3-step training method for carving/constructing 3D ear framework.[13] Step 1 is to learn the 3D shape of the ear framework by sculpting a 3D framework out of a potato. This practice model was started by Brent,[3] and I modified it; I use a precise ear template as a guide to learn the importance of the preciseness for the framework. Step 2 is to learn the assembly process of 5 components of the 3D ear framework. Step 3 is to learn how to transform the rib cartilage shape into a 3D ear framework. Precise copy of rib cartilage (6–9), and precise ear template makes the simulation surgery very realistic to the clinical situation.

If surgeons work at a pediatric hospital, human rib cartilage may be available, removed and disposed of after pectus excavatum surgery (Step 4) (**Fig. 21**).

SUMMARY

Although the Nagata technique is technically demanding, if the technique is mastered, the surgeon can produce satisfactory long-term outcomes with minimal complications. The key is "do not perform clinical cases until the surgeon becomes absolutely confident about 3D fame-carving techniques." Basic reconstructive skills, such as delicate skin flap preparation, skin harvesting, and harvesting rib cartilage without perichondrium, are also a must. It is important to remember that microtia patients have only one best chance for optimal outcome. Simulation surgery proposed by the author is an effective "self-training method" to master 3D framework construct.

REFERENCES

1. Tanzer RC. Total reconstruction of the external ear. Plast Reconstr Surg 1959;23:1.
2. Tanzer RC. Congenital deformities of the auricle. In: Converse JM, editor. Reconstructive plastic surgery. Philadelphia: W.B. Saunders Company; 1964. p. 1073.
3. Brent BD. Reconstruction of the ear. In: Neligan PC, editor. Plastic surgery. 3rd edition. Philadelphia: Elsevier Saunders; 2013. p. 187–225.
4. Nagata S. The modification stages involved in the total reconstruction of the auricle: part I. The modification in the grafting of the three-dimensional costal cartilage framework (3-D frame) for the lobule type microtia. Plast Reconstr Surg 1994;93: 221–30.
5. Nagata S. The modification stages involved in the total reconstruction of the auricle: part II. The modification in the grafting of the three-dimensional costal cartilage framework (3-D frame) for the concha type microtia. Plast Reconstr Surg 1994; 93:231–42.
6. Nagata S. The modification stages involved in the total reconstruction of the auricle: part III. The modification in the grafting of the three-dimensional costal cartilage framework (3-D frame) for the small concha type microtia. Plast Reconstr Surg 1994;93: 243–53.
7. Tolleth H. Concepts for the plastic surgeon from art and sculpture. Clin Plast Surg 1987;14(4):585–98.
8. Tolleth H. Artistic anatomy, dimensions, and proportions of the external ear. Clin Plast Surg 1978;5(3): 337. Saunders.
9. Farkas LG. Anthropometry of the normal and defective ear. Clin Plast Surg 1990;17(2):213–21.

10. Yamada A, Ueda K, Harada T. Aesthetic curve analysis of the normal auricle: development of normal ear templates and its clinical application for total auricular reconstruction. J Plast Surg (Japanese) 2011;54(3):251–9.

11. Kawanabe Y, Nagata S. A new method of costal cartilage harvest for total auricular reconstruction: part II. Evaluation and analysis of the regenerated costal cartilage. Plast Reconstr Surg 2007;119(1):308–15.

12. Brent B, Byrd HS. Secondary ear reconstruction with cartilage graft covered by axial, random, and free flaps of temporoparietal fascia. Plast Reconstr Surg 1983;72:141.

13. Yamada A, Imai K, Fujimoto T, et al. New training method of creating ear framework by using precise copy of costal cartilage. J Craniofac Surg 2009; 20(3):899–902.

Pediatric Microtia Reconstruction with Autologous Rib
Personal Experience and Technique with 1000 Pediatric Patients with Microtia

Arturo Bonilla, MD

KEYWORDS

- Pediatric • Microtia reconstruction • Autologous rib • Technique

KEY POINTS

- Reconstruction of the microtic ear is one of the most challenging, yet gratifying surgical experiences.
- Careful planning, attention to detail, and conservative tissue management are necessary for excellent results.
- Technologies continue to evolve; with the advancement of cartilage tissue engineering, the future of ear reconstruction is very promising.

INTRODUCTION

Microtia is the most common major congenital malformation of the ear. It is usually accompanied with atresia or lack of an ear canal. Because of the multiple specialties that should be involved in the management of a child with microtia and atresia, it is of utmost importance to begin this as soon as the child is born. These specialists include the pediatrician[1]; microtia surgeon; geneticist; ear, nose, and throat surgeon; audiologist; and speech and language therapists. If available, craniofacial teams are excellent for evaluating and managing microtia and atresia for these children.

Although the numbers may vary, microtia occurs in 1 in 1000 to 1 in 5800 to 8000 births.[2] It usually occurs more often in boys and on the right side. Associated malformations may occur in children with microtia, such as hemifacial macrosomia, facial nerve weakness, urogenital defects, and cardiac and spine defects. Associated syndromes, such as Goldenhar syndrome and Treacher-Collins syndrome, very often have microtia and atresia.[3] Fortunately, the cochlear function is usually normal despite having a microtia and atresia on either side.[4]

Although the absolute cause of microtia and atresia are unknown, the most common theory is the ischemia or obliteration of the stapedial artery. Genetic studies are being actively performed and may provide further clues. Known drugs, such as thalidomide and isotretinoin, have been described in the past.

CLASSIFICATION

Microtia is classified into 4 grades (**Fig. 1**):

Grade 1: The ear is slightly smaller than normal but retains most of the anatomic characteristics of the normal ear. Although atresia can be present, there is usually an external auditory canal.

Grade 2: The ear is even smaller and is less developed than grade 1. Part of the helix may be

The author has nothing to disclose.
Microtia–Congenital, Ear Deformity Institute, 9502 Huebner Road, Suite 301, San Antonio, TX 78240
E-mail address: doctorbonilla@microtia.net

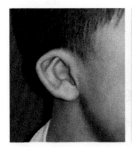 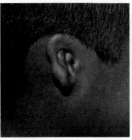 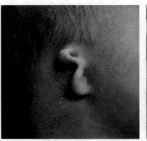 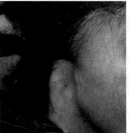

Fig. 1. Grade 1, 2, 3, and 4 microtia.

developed. The triangular fossa, scaphae, and antihelix are less developed. Atresia may or may not be present.

Grade 3 or classic: This grade is the most common type of microtia. It is usually a vertical remnant of skin consisting of a superior part that is made up of disorganized cartilage and an inferior part that is the displaced earlobe. Atresia is almost always associated with this type of microtia.

Grade 4 or anotia: There is complete absence of an outer ear structure. Atresia is almost always associated with anotia.

EVALUATION AND MANAGEMENT

The most optimal time to consult on a child with microtia is before the child leaves the hospital. This time would also be ideal to speak with the parents of the child. There is usually much parental stress involved because of the uncertainty of the management. It is common for parents to feel guilty and a source of the cause of their child with microtia. Other common parental concerns include hearing loss, speech and language delays, learning disabilities, future bullying, cost or coverage of surgeries, and many more. Because of these uncertainties and worries, it is critical to consult with the parents early in order to educate them and provide them with realistic expectations. Newborn hearing screenings are normally performed before the patients' discharge from the hospital. Before discharge, there should be a plan in place to perform audiologic testing. If a child is affected only on one side (unilateral) and the normal ear has normal hearing, there is more time to visit all of the specialists with patience. If a child is affected on both sides (bilateral), then it is crucial to perform earlier brainstem auditory-evoked response testing in order to supply the child with a bone-conduction headband.

Evaluation by the microtia specialist is of utmost importance. The microtia surgeon can advise the family on all of the options, including observation, rib cartilage, porous polyethylene, and prosthetics. The timing of surgical interventions varies depending on the technique and the surgeon, so it is important to cover all of these options early on. In addition, the various techniques in auditory management need to be coordinated with the microtia surgeon in order to optimize the timing of the hearing correction.

TIMING OF AUTOLOGOUS CARTILAGE RECONSTRUCTION

Although some cartilage surgeons prefer to wait until the child is approximately 9 to 10 years of age, it is very common to begin the auricular reconstruction with costal cartilage around 6 to 7 years of age. Experience and judgment of timing is critical because if a child's surgery is started too early and the child is too small, there may not be enough cartilage to make an adequate-sized ear compared with the normal side. In the author's experience, approximately 45 to 47 in of height has been adequate to begin the reconstruction as long as the normal ear is not too large. If the child is too small or the normal ear is rather large, then the surgery is delayed until everything is optimized. In addition, the author strongly thinks that the child should be aware and have some understanding and decision-making in this process.

In the past, surgical reconstruction on children who had bilateral microtia and atresia was begun at 4 years of age because there was not a normal-sized ear to compare. Because of the excellent advances in hearing management, the author prefers to wait until the child is 6 to 7 years of age with bilateral microtia as well.

Certain techniques prefer external auditory canal surgery before the outer ear surgery, whereas others, such as the cartilage technique, prefer the external auditory canal surgery to always follow the outer ear surgery. Cartilage surgeons prefer elastic, virgin skin in order to provide the best skin coverage of the cartilaginous framework. If there is much scar before the microtia surgery, the skin is not as elastic and the final outcome may not be optimal.

The author's technique involves 3 surgical stages divided every 2 months. Once the surgery is initiated, most ears are completed in 4 months. If the child is affected bilaterally, then the surgical stages are combined and 4 stages are performed over a span of about 6 months.

THE FIRST SURGICAL STAGE (CARTILAGE HARVESTING FROM RIB CAVITY)
First-Stage Introduction

The author's surgical technique is a modification from the classic Brent technique.[5] If the child is of adequate size, the first stage is begun. Excellent understanding of the 3-dimensional landmarks of the ear will give the surgeon the most tools to perform a successful surgery. During the first stage, the synchondrosis of ribs 6 and 7 as well as the cartilaginous part of rib 8 are harvested (**Fig. 2**). In order to avoid a chest wall deformity, the least amount of rib cartilage is harvested that will fully build the size of the new ear compared with the contralateral ear. If much cartilage is removed and unused parts discarded, then the unnecessary removal of cartilage can result in an increased chance of a chest wall deformity. If part of the perichondrium on the undersurface of the ribs is preserved, there will be less chance of a deformity. If there is a low hairline, laser hair

removal may be performed before the surgical reconstruction.[6] A crescent of hair-bearing scalp may also be excised and covered with a skin graft.[7]

First-Stage Technique

The first stage is performed under general anesthesia. Although the author initially used assistant surgeons, the efficiency of a one-surgeon approach has sped up the first stage to approximately 2.0 to 2.5 hours. A diagonal incision with a No. 15 scalpel (approximately 2.0–2.5 cm) is made over the areas of ribs 6, 7, and 8 on the contralateral chest wall (**Fig. 3**).

A special contact laser is used to limit the thermal injury and decrease the chance of bleeding. The subcutaneous fat is then incised with the contact laser down to the level of the rectus muscle. The rectus muscle is divided with the contact laser using a horizontal technique until ribs 6, 7, and 8 are easily visualized. At this point, the x-ray template that had been used to mark the size of the normal ear and sterilized is now placed over the ribs to be removed (**Fig. 4**). The ribs to be removed are marked with a sterile marker. The skin hooks are then used to retract the eighth rib. Using the contact laser, the soft tissue around the rib is carefully excised with attention to angle the laser tip away from the pulmonary cavity. Once the eighth rib is excised, it is placed in a solution of normal saline/antibiotic solution. The skin hooks are then used to retract the synchondrosis of the sixth and seventh rib. In a similar fashion, the rib is excised with the contact laser with care to leave some perichondrium on the undersurface of the rib to avoid a chest wall deformity. Once removed, the synchondrosis of ribs 6 and 7 are placed in the

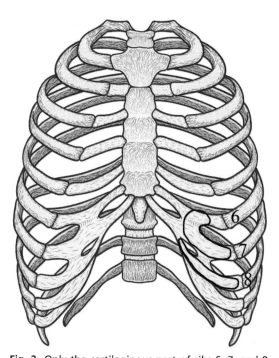

Fig. 2. Only the cartilaginous part of ribs 6, 7, and 8 are harvested. The eighth rib forms the helix, and the synchondrosis of ribs 6 and 7 forms the main base of the new ear.

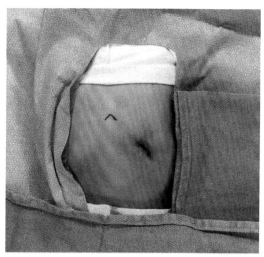

Fig. 3. A small, diagonal chest incision is performed on the contralateral side. The incision is usually 2.0 to 2.5 cm.

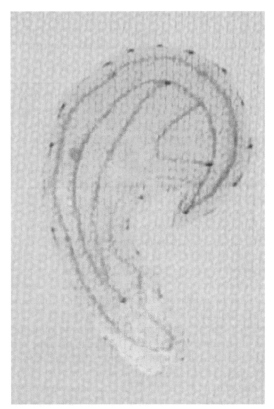

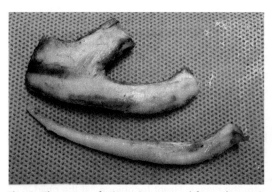

Fig. 6. The extrasoft tissue is removed from the cartilage preserving the perichondrium.

Fig. 4. An x-ray template is used to measure the size and landmarks of the contralateral ear. If patients have bilateral microtia, the size and shape may be performed freehand. The x-ray template is then sterilized and used intraoperatively to remove only the needed cartilage.

same normal saline/antibiotic solution (**Fig. 5**). The soft tissue is then removed from the ribs while maintaining as much perichondrium as possible (**Fig. 6**). A Blake drain is placed under the muscle

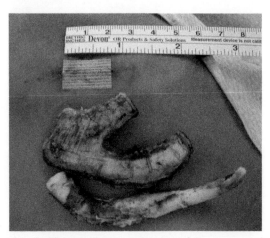

Fig. 5. The cartilage was successfully harvested through a 2-cm incision.

layer and attached to the skin with a 4-0 Prolene (Ethicon, Somerville, NJ) suture. The muscle layer is closed with interrupted 4-0 Mersilene (Ethicon) sutures. The soft tissue layer is also closed with 4-0 Mersilene sutures. The skin is closed with a subcuticular 5-0 Vicryl (Ethicon) suture. Dermabond (Ethicon) is then placed over the skin, and Steri-Strips (3M, St Paul, MN) are then placed.

The ribs are then taken to a sterile side table for sculpting. During this time, the anesthesiologist turns patients to the side and performs an epidural injection so that patients may be pain free immediately postoperatively.

The perichondrium on one side of the eighth rib is thinned in order to force a curve of the future helix. Care must be taken to avoid removing too much cartilage to avoid buckling or resorption. The x-ray template is then placed over the synchondrosis, and the cartilage is marked. The No. 15 scalpel is then used to sculpt the shape of the synchondrosis to match the shape of the contralateral ear. A No. 6 dermal punch is used to deepen the area of the scaphae and the triangular fossa according to the x-ray template. A No. 4 dermal punch is then used to make holes in the scaphae in order to allow suction of the skin over the framework when suction is attached. The eighth rib (helix) is placed over the sixth and seventh (synchondrosis) and secured with interrupted 4-0 clear nylon sutures with the knots on the undersurface of the ear (**Fig. 7**). In addition, a small extra piece of cartilage is excised to form the future tragus[8] by suturing it to the helical root superiorly and the lower framework inferiorly with a 4-0 clear nylon suture. Once this is performed, the size of the new cartilaginous framework is confirmed with the x-ray template (**Fig. 8**).

The microtic ear is now prepped and draped in a sterile fashion. The ear marking that had been drawn preoperatively is then injected with local

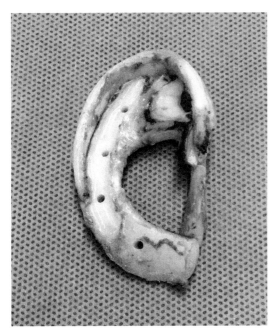

Fig. 7. This image demonstrates the sculpted cartilaginous framework, including the tragus. Small holes are placed through the scaphae to improve the suction of the skin on the cartilage.

anesthetic (**Fig. 9**). An incision is made just anterior to the microtic skin vestige (**Fig. 10**). The skin is undermined with a tenotomy scissor while preserving the subdermal plexus. The elevation continues several millimeters past the marking in order to provide enough elasticity over the helix. The vestigial cartilage is then carefully excised with careful attention to avoid button-holing the

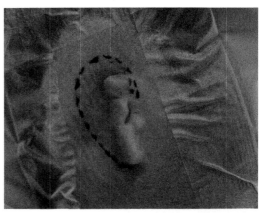

Fig. 9. The location of the ear is marked preoperatively.

skin. The cartilaginous framework is placed under the skin pocket, and a Blake drain is placed under the framework and placed on suction. Once the skin is closed with a running 6-0 Prolene suture, the skin very nicely suctions over the cartilaginous framework (**Fig. 11**). This draping of the skin over the cartilage is crucial to provide an adequate blood supply. It is important to assure that a preauricular sinus is not present because an unnoticed sinus tract may be the nidus for a future infection with possible resorption of the cartilage. If a sinus tract is present, it is crucial to excise this either during the first-stage surgery or ideally before this stage (**Fig. 12**). A sterile ear cup is placed to protect the ear from trauma. The first stage is now complete. Patients are placed on 23-hour observation and discharged the following morning. One week later, the drains are

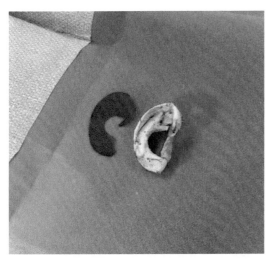

Fig. 8. The cartilaginous framework is placed next to the x-ray template to check for the appropriate size before insertion under the skin pocket.

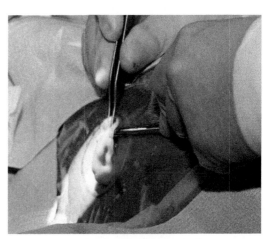

Fig. 10. A small vertical incision is made anterior to the microtic vestige, and the skin is undermined while preserving the subdermal plexus. The vestigial cartilage is removed.

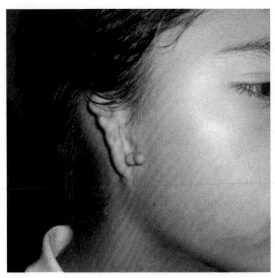
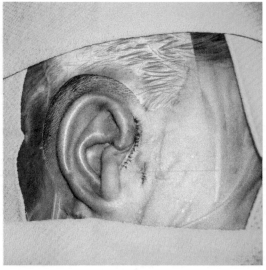

Fig. 11. Preoperative and intraoperative results after the first stage.

removed; the following week, the sutures are removed (**Fig. 13**).

THE SECOND SURGICAL STAGE (FORMATION OF THE EARLOBE AND DEEPENING OF THE CONCHAL BASE)
Second-Stage Introduction

The second stage is an outpatient procedure that takes approximately 45 minutes. It is performed approximately 2 months after the first stage. During this stage, the lower microtic vestige (lobule) is transposed posteriorly to its final position and the conchal bowl is then deepened in preparation for a possible ear canal surgery.

Second-Stage Technique

An incision is made anterior to the microtic skin vestige and directed superiorly over the vestige and brought down posterior to the vestige preserving the inferior pedicle. A z-plasty is then performed. Using a tenotomy scissor, a pocket is made in the actual lobule to house the inferior cartilaginous framework. Approximately 1 cm of the lower cartilaginous framework is exposed

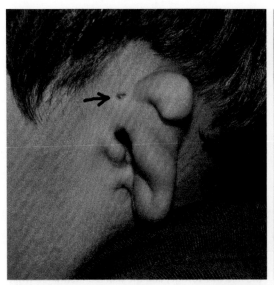
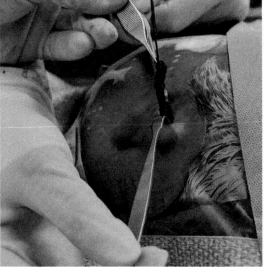

Fig. 12. Small pits around the ear need to be examined in order to avoid missing a preauricular sinus tract, which can lead to future infection. In this case, a tract was located and removed before the first-stage reconstruction.

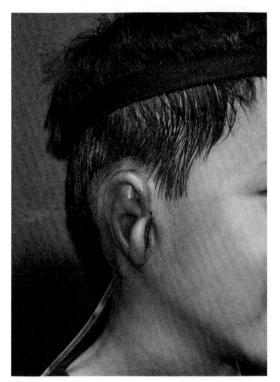

Fig. 13. The drain is removed 1 week after the first stage. Notice the definition and natural color of the skin.

while preserving the perichondrium. This lower framework is placed into the skin pocket to provide lifelong inferior to superior elongation of the ear. The extra superior skin of the remnant is then removed as a full-thickness skin graft and placed in normal saline/antibiotic solution. The soft tissue of the conchal area is excised and deepened to the level of the tragal cartilage that was sculpted during the first stage. The full-thickness skin graft is then placed into the

conchal base and sutured with 5-0 chromic sutures.

The remaining skin of the lobule is closed with either 6-0 Prolene sutures or interrupted 5-0 chromic sutures depending on the tightness of the skin. Antibiotic ointment is then placed over the wound, and a sterile ear cup is placed to protect the ear from trauma. The second stage is now complete. **Figs. 14–16** show the transposition of the lobule to its final position.

THE THIRD SURGICAL STAGE (ELEVATION OF THE EAR): HYBRID APPROACH

The third and final stage is an outpatient procedure that takes approximately 2 hours. Historically, cartilage reconstructions have lacked ear protrusion. Attempts have been made to bank an extra rib and use this rib to increase the protrusion. Resorption still occurred. The author developed a new approach. During this stage, the ear is elevated and a hybrid approach using a specially made wedge of polyethylene is inserted under the ear to give the ear protrusion and avoid a flat ear that has haunted cartilage surgeons for decades. The author devised this hybrid technique many years ago to give the ear more elevation on the undersurface while preserving the full cartilaginous outer ear.

Third-Stage Technique

A marking is made 3 mm outside the boundary of the cartilaginous framework (**Fig. 17**). In addition, an elliptical area in the contralateral inguinal area that is the height of the ear framework is also marked. The markings are infiltrated with local anesthetic. The ear all the way down to the inguinal area is prepped and draped. A No. 15 scalpel is used to make an incision on the outer boundary of the helix from the superior ear all the way

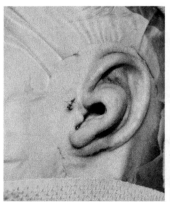
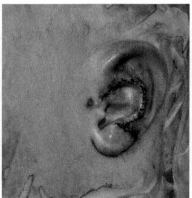
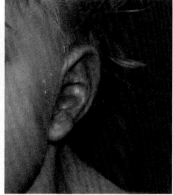

Fig. 14. The second-stage earlobe transposition.

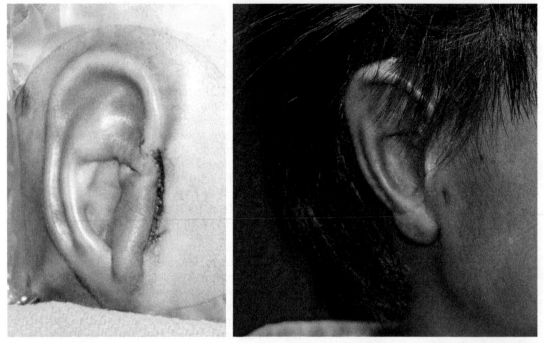

Fig. 15. The second-stage preoperative and postoperative results. The lower part of the cartilaginous framework is inserted into a pocket within the lobule.

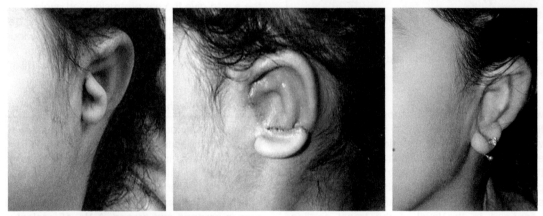

Fig. 16. The second-stage earlobe transposition.

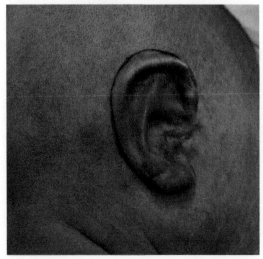

Fig. 17. Markings before the third-stage elevation procedure.

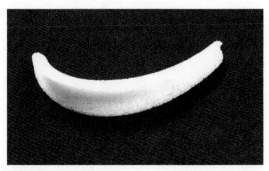

Fig. 18. A custom-designed polyethylene wedge is used to give the ear excellent protrusion.

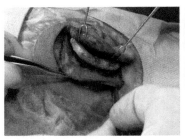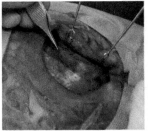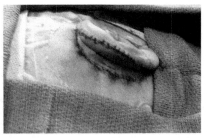

Fig. 19. The ear is elevated during the third stage, and an occipital flap is used to cover the polyethylene wedge. A full-thickness skin graft harvested from the inguinal area is then placed.

down to the lobule. A polyethylene wedge implant is placed in sterile betadine solution preoperatively (**Fig. 18**). One-half of the cartilaginous framework is undermined with a tenotomy scissor. The posterior scalp is then undermined approximately 3 cm preserving an anterior-based occipital flap. At this point, the wedge implant is fitted in the postauricular sulcus and trimmed to fit the undersurface of the ear as well as to provide the same protrusion as the contralateral ear. A contralateral otoplasty is performed if that ear protrudes too much. An occipital based flap is then raised to completely cover the wedge implant. Once there is adequate coverage, the flap is sutured to the undersurface of the cartilaginous framework with interrupted 4-0 Mersilene sutures. The posterior scalp is then advanced anteriorly and secured with the mastoid periosteum with interrupted 4-0 Mersilene sutures (**Fig. 19**). At this point, a No. 15 scalpel is used to incise the elliptical-shaped markings of the contralateral inguinal area. A full-thickness skin graft is

then harvested and placed in normal saline/antibiotic solution. The soft tissue of the inguinal wound is closed with interrupted 4-0 Mersilene sutures. The skin is closed with a running 4-0 Vicryl suture. Dermabond is placed and Steri-Strips are applied. A pressure dressing is then placed. The full-thickness skin graft is placed over the new retroauricular sulcus, and the skin edges are closed with interrupted 5-0 chromic sutures. The base of the skin graft is secured to the base of the retroauricular sulcus with 5-0 chromic sutures. Antibiotic ointment is then applied to the skin graft, and a sterile sponge is placed over the skin graft and secured with mild pressure using 4-0 Prolene sutures (**Fig. 20**). This step is performed to avoid a seroma under the skin graft. **Fig. 21** demonstrates a patient after the elevation procedure. **Fig. 22**

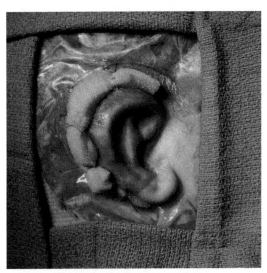

Fig. 20. A sterile sponge is placed with mild pressure to avoid a seroma or hematoma under the full-thickness skin graft.

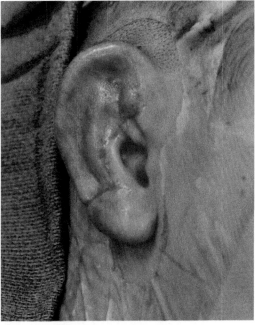

Fig. 21. Appearance of the ear after the third-stage elevation procedure.

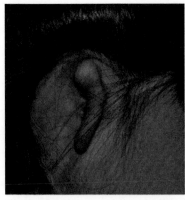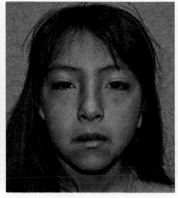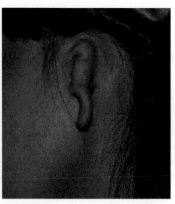

Fig. 22. Preoperative appearance of a patient with bilateral microtia before the third-stage elevation procedure.

demonstrates a patient with bilateral microtia preoperatively. **Fig. 23** shows the patient in **Fig. 22** after the third-stage elevation procedure. **Fig. 24** demonstrates the intraoperative and postoperative appearance of a child with microtia after the elevation stage.

Figs. 25–27 demonstrate the preoperative and postoperative results of patients using the author's 3 stage technique.

COMPLICATIONS

Complications using the autologous cartilage technique are relatively rare. It is important to adequately raise the appropriate thickness of the skin pocket during the first stage in order to avoid ischemia of the skin, but raising a skin pocket that is too thick may result in an ear with decreased definition. Using the contact laser system, bleeding averages 5 to 10 mL during the entire first stage and less during the subsequent stages. If there is not adequate hemostasis intraoperatively or if there is postoperative trauma, a hematoma may occur that could require surgical evacuation. Infection is also rare because of the utilization of the patients' own living tissues. With careful dissection, the risk of pneumothorax during the cartilage harvesting is rare. The most common risk regardless of the technique is most likely a nonaesthetically pleasing ear, albeit a rare occurrence if performed by an experienced surgeon.

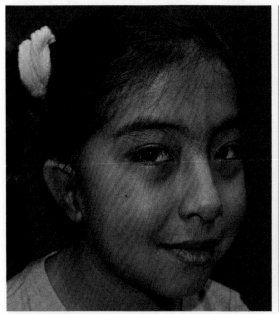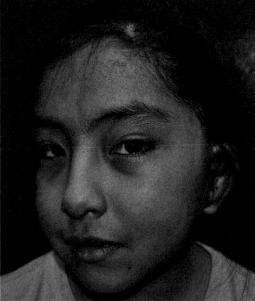

Fig. 23. Postoperative appearance of the patient from **Fig. 22** after the third-stage elevation procedure.

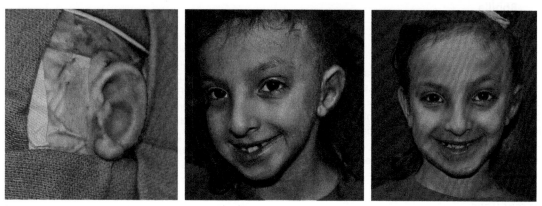

Fig. 24. Intraoperative and postoperative appearance of a patient after the third-stage elevation procedure.

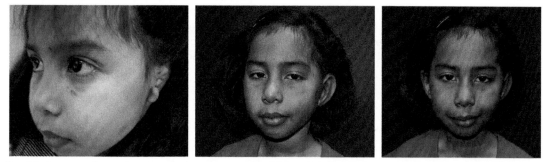

Fig. 25. Preoperative and postoperative pictures of a child with left-sided grade 3 microtia and atresia.

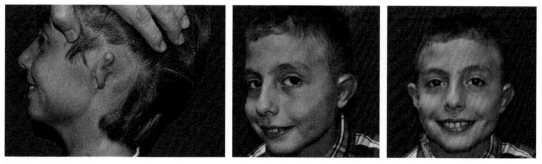

Fig. 26. Preoperative and postoperative pictures of a child with left-sided grade 3 microtia and atresia.

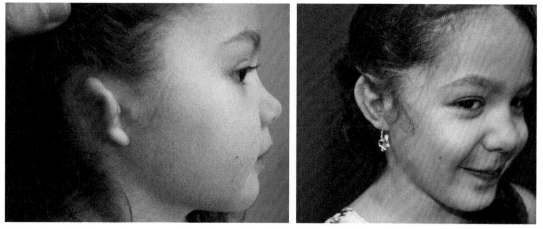

Fig. 27. Preoperative and postoperative pictures of a child with right-sided grade 3 microtia and atresia.

SUMMARY

Reconstruction of the microtic ear is one of the most challenging, yet gratifying surgical experiences. Careful planning, attention to detail, and conservative tissue management is necessary for excellent results. Technologies continue to evolve; with the advancement of cartilage tissue engineering, the future of ear reconstruction is very promising.

REFERENCES

1. Brent B. The pediatrician's role in caring for patients with congenital microtia and atresia. Pediatr Ann 1999;28:374.

2. Jahrsdoerfer RA, Hall JW. Congenital atresia of the ear. Laryngoscope 1978;88(suppl 13):1.

3. Brent B. Microtia repair with rib cartilage grafts: a review of personal experience with 1000 cases. Clin Plast Surg 2002;29:257–71.

4. Jahrsdoerfer RA, Cole RR, Gray LC. Advances in congenital aural atresia. In: Advances in otolaryngology – head and neck surgery. St. Louis (France): Mosby; 1991. p. 1–15.

5. Brent B. Auricular repair with autogenous rib cartilage grafts: two decades of experience with 600 cases. Plast Reconstr Surg 1992;90:355–74.

6. Wheeland RG. Laser-assisted hair removal. Dermatol Clin 1997;15:469.

7. Eavey RD. Microtia repair: creation of a functional postauricular sulcus. Otolaryngol Head Neck Surg 1999;120:789.

8. Bonilla JA, Yellon RF. Surgical management of microtia and congenital aural atresia. Pediatric otolaryngology. 4th edition. 2003. p. 420–40.

Auricular Reconstruction Using Porous Polyethylene Implant Technique

Scott Stephan, MD[a],*, John Reinisch, MD[b]

KEYWORDS

- Auricular reconstruction • Porous polyethylene • Implant • Ear

KEY POINTS

- Porous high-density polyethylene as an alloplast in microtia reconstruction offers an excellent framework for auricular reconstruction.
- Advantages include earlier reconstruction, fewer procedures, avoidance of donor site morbidity, shorter learning curve, and improved size and contour match.
- Results ultimately depend on soft tissue envelope, and choice of technique is best decided according to surgeon expertise and patient preference.

INTRODUCTION

Creation of an external ear remains one of the most challenging dilemmas for reconstructive surgeons. Between the thin soft tissue envelope surrounding an intricate, flexible framework projecting off the mastoid, success in recreating native anatomy depends as much on the patient's soft tissue characteristics as it does on surgical technique.

The choice of material for creating the architecture and framework of the ear has long been a topic of debate and continues to evolve. Staged autologous cartilage reconstruction remains the most widely used technique in microtia repair,[1] but many surgeons have turned to alloplasts to avoid donor site morbidity, begin reconstruction at an earlier age, reduce the number of total surgeries, increase the predictability of their results, improve on the inherent structural limitations of autologous rib, and to tailor to individual patients' needs (ie, low-lying hairline, bilateral microtia). This article broadly discusses the considerations for alloplast-based ear reconstruction, details a series of evolving technical advancements, and expands on the description of the surgical procedure outlined in the authors' previous work.[2]

AURICULAR ALLOPLASTS

The ideal alloplast for auricular reconstruction would be cost-effective, safely implantable, resistant to infection and repeated trauma, and be easily customized to approximate the contralateral native ear.

Since 1891, more than 40 different framework materials have been described in the ear, including alloplasts such as ivory, wire mesh, nylon, and silicone.[3,4] Silicone was initially viewed as a promising prospect, particularly for its ability to mimic

Disclosure: The authors have nothing to disclose.
[a] Department of Otolaryngology, Head and Neck Surgery, Vanderbilt University Medical Center, 7th Floor Medical Center East, South Tower, 1211 Medical Center Drive, Nashville, TN 37232, USA; [b] Department of Surgery, University of Southern California, 1450 San Pablo Street, Healthcare Consultation Center 4 Suite 6200, Los Angeles, CA 90089, USA
* Corresponding author.
E-mail address: Stephan@vanderbilt.edu

the flexibility and structure of native auricular cartilage, but a high extrusion rate when placed under thin skin flaps was ultimately problematic.[5]

First described for partial auricular reconstruction by Berghaus and colleagues[19] in 1983, porous high-density polyethylene (pHDPE), originally marketed as Medpor (Stryker, Kalamazoo, MI) has a long record of successful, safe use as an implantable framework. Other companies now offer similar pHDPE ear implants, such as Omnipore (Matrix Surgical USA, Atlanta, GA) and Su-Por (Poriferous, Newnan, GA). pHDPE is a modestly flexible, biocompatible material made of high-density polyethylene with interconnected pores (100–200 µm diameter) that show structural stability and the ability to support soft tissue ingrowth.[6,7] As a porous material, this facilitates collagen deposition and vascular ingrowth, which in turn protects against extrusion and infection, and allows systemic drug delivery to the implant.[8] Structurally, pHDPE is robust enough to withstand the repeated microtrauma expected of an ear, but is easily shapeable with a scalpel, and separate pieces may be soldered together with high-temperature cautery. The authors' experience with customization with drill technique is reviewed later.

The basic paradigm for microtia reconstruction using a pHDPE implant involves implantation of a fused two-piece framework, completely covered with a large temporoparietal fascia (TPF) flap and resurfaced with a mixture of skin grafts and local flaps. This procedure has been described as both single stage[5] and multistage.[4,9–11]

CONSIDERATIONS FOR HIGH-DENSITY POROUS POLYETHYLENE

One advantage of alloplast reconstruction is the avoidance of a chest wall donor site. Because the quantity and quality of the patient's rib cartilage is not a factor, patients do not need to wait for chest wall maturity for costal cartilage harvest, and may undergo reconstruction at an earlier age. The youngest child implanted in the authors' experience was 2.5 years old, with preferred timing between 3 and 6 years of age. pHDPE is available as a preformed 2-piece implant, and a straightforward technique allows a shorter learning curve for new surgeons. Modern modifications to the procedure have resulted in comparable complication rates with autologous cartilage, and cosmetic outcomes can be excellent in experienced hands.[4,12] Microtia reconstruction with porous polyethylene may be performed after or at the same time as canal atresia surgery if the patient is deemed a suitable candidate for canalplasty.

Thus, patients can have their atresia and microtia reconstructions completed in a single stage before entering primary school, which is an important period of cognitive awareness and self-concept.[13–15] There are also aesthetic and technical considerations as to why pHDPE auricular reconstruction is better earlier than later in the authors' experience: the TPF flap used to cover the implant is the blood supply to the overlying hair follicles and becomes thicker as the child approaches late adolescence to teenage years, perhaps as a factor of increased hair density and caliber with puberty. When done at an early age, the TPF is thin and more pliable, allowing it to easily contour to the architecture of the implant under negative pressure, yielding superior detail. There is significantly less bleeding and better visualization of surgical planes in younger children than in adolescents and adults. Also, the dermal layer of the harvested full-thickness skin grafts used to cover the TPF flap is also inherently thinner.

Although salvage surgery using autologous rib with adjunctive procedures has been described,[16,17] it is not common and the outcomes are widely variable. In contrast, the pHDPE implant–based approach is versatile; it serves as an excellent primary option in many cases or can be used as salvage surgery after failed autologous rib, burn cases, auricular avulsion, or situations of significant scarring of the mastoid skin area, provided that a well-vascularized fascial flap is still available for framework coverage.

TECHNIQUE

The authors' reconstructive approach is described later, adapted from the single-stage technique first described by the senior author and modified over the years to the current iteration.[3,5] The emphasis is on microtia reconstruction, but the principles remain generalized for auricular reconstruction broadly.

PREP

The patient is orotracheally intubated and the bed rotated 180°. Hair over the temporoparietal area on the surgical side is shaved to allow proper Doppler identification of the vascular anatomy. The course of the superficial temporal artery is mapped using vascular Doppler and a permanent skin marker. The anterior and posterior branches of the superficial temporal artery (STA) are marked and, if possible, any superior anastomosing arcade between the 2 ends distally (Fig. 1).

It can be helpful to identify the main trunk of the STA as it courses near the auricular remnant. In

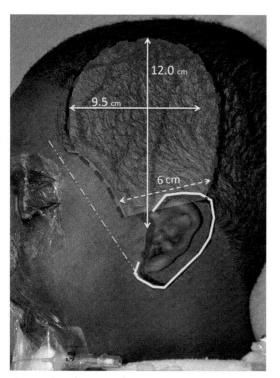

Fig. 1. Identification of landmarks and flap design. Yellow lines indicate skin incisions. Vertical dimension of the TPF flap is measured from the proposed superior border of the neo-external auditory canal extending vertically toward the vertex of the scalp. The anterior/posterior dimension is slightly narrower, extending to the temporal hairline to incorporate the anterior branch of the STA (demarcated in red). The base of the TPF flap is kept wide to maintain venous drainage in the mastoid region. (*From* Owen S, Wang T, Stephan S. Alloplastic reconstruction of the microtic ear. Operat Tech Otolaryngol Head Neck Surg 2017;28(2):98; with permission.)

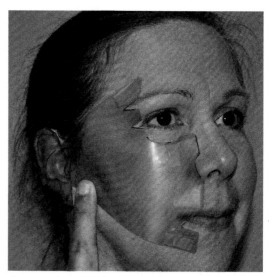

Fig. 2. Radiograph film tailored to dimensions of the contralateral ear with surface landmarks of the lateral brow, lateral canthus, malar-orbital groove, alar-facial groove, and oral commissure used to orient the new ear on the opposite side with respect to location and axis. Intra-auricular details such as the superior and inferior crura as well as the shape of the conchal bowl are cut as single lines through the film.

severe cases of microtia, the vessel can originate from the post-auricular artery rather than being the terminal branch of the external cartodi vessel. In these cases the vessel begins behind the lobe and courses underneath the microtic cartilage putting the vessel in danger during removal of the cartilage remnant.

The anticipated course of the frontal branch of the facial nerve is also delineated using the Pitanguy line principle, using the mastoid tip as the inferior point of reference in place of the lobule.

Using a piece of radiograph film (or the clear plastic guard from a surgical face mask), the position and size of the contralateral normal ear are marked relative to the oral commissure, nasal alar groove, orbitomalar groove, lateral canthus, and lateral brow **Fig. 2**. The radiograph film can be sterilized for later use on the field, or the plastic mask sheet can be covered by sterile translucent dressings. The dimensions of the new ear are based on the contralateral normal ear, taking into consideration the patient's age at the time of surgery and anticipated future growth. In addition, notes are taken of specific details and unique features found on the normal ear that will be customized during the molding and soldering of the implant later in the procedure.

Careful preoperative assessment of the patient's age, contralateral ear dimensions in the setting of unilateral microtia, as well as the dimensions of their gender-matched parent's ear are essential to achieving symmetry between the reconstructed pHDPE ear and the normal ear. The pHDPE will not increase in size so an adult-sized ear must be created at the time of surgery. In a forensic study of normative data for ear growth in more than 800 patients, at 4 to 5 years of age, ear vertical length was approximately 90% (girls) and 84% to 86% (boys) of the relevant values recorded in individuals 18 to 30 years old.[18] Therefore, adding a 10% to 15% increase in height from the contralateral ear in a 4-year-old patient (about 5–7 mm) is a reasonable estimation; using dimensions from the parents can also be a double check (**Fig. 3**). A case example of a boy 3 years and 2 months old who underwent pHDPE microtia reconstruction with modest adjustment in size for future growth shows the ability to accurately compensate for this dynamic even in very young patients (**Fig. 4**).

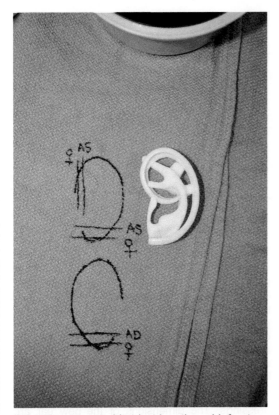

Fig. 3. For a 7-year-old girl with unilateral left microtia reconstruction, measurements of the normal right ear (AD) as well as that of her mother's right ear are shown at the bottom of the image. Using this information, the proposed left ear (AS) size is then designed and the pHDPE implant customized to what will be her predicted adult-sized ear.

Likewise, a perfectly symmetric ear that is moderately malpositioned may be an even greater disfigurement and distraction than the original

microtia. Of the facial landmarks used for orientation, the lateral brow, lateral canthus, malar-orbital groove, and alar groove are the most trustworthy in patients with some degree of craniofacial microsomia, because the first and second branchial arch malformations disproportionately affect the lower facial skeleton. The patient's eyes, nose, and mouth are kept visible but covered with an occlusive transparent dressing to remain out of the sterile field. The head is prepped with betadine solution, and the auricular remnant, incisions, and skin graft donor sites injected with local anesthetic.

The scalp incisions used to approach the TPF flap elevation are varied, with multiple approaches described. The authors favor elevation of the flap entirely from below, using only the incision in the postauricular area of the microtic ear corresponding with the position of the new helical rim. This incision is made on the postauricular component of the portion of the ear that is present (**Fig. 5**). In patients with low-set hairlines, up to a third or half of this incision along its superior margin may be in hair-bearing skin. Whatever component of the anteriorly based mastoid skin flap contains hair is discarded. Therefore, the surgeon does not have to compromise either the placement of the implant or the final aesthetics of a hairy ear based on the patient's preoperative mastoid hairline position. To improve exposure, a curvilinear horizontal incision over the superior portion of the TPF flap can be added; this additional incision can help visualize the distal most portion of the anterior branch as it travels just posterior to the frontal branch of facial nerve. It can also be helpful in harvesting the distal flap to obtain the recommended length. These two approaches allow adequate access to elevate a wide TPF flap with a lighted retractor or head light.

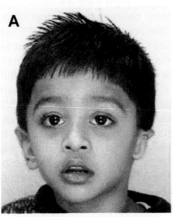
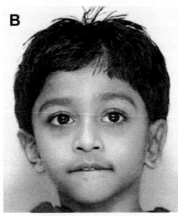
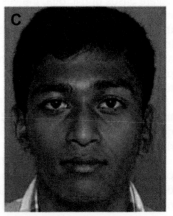

Fig. 4. (*A*) Child seen before left ear reconstruction at 3 years and 2 months; (*B*) 10 months after left ear reconstruction with modest adjust in vertical height; (*C*) same patient see at 20 years of age with good interaural height symmetry. (*From* Reinisch J. Ear reconstruction in young children. Facial Plast Surg 2015;31:602; with permission.)

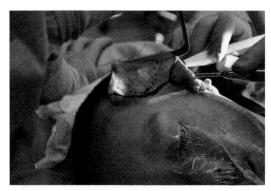

Fig. 5. Elevation of the TPF flap is done through the postauricular incision only using needle tip electrocautery and a headlight or lighted retractor.

Other approaches include a Y incision extending superiorly from the mastoid area, as well as a large Z to expose the TPF. Each of these allow much better visualization and access to the fascia but carry the risk of patchy alopecia near incisional bifurcations or the apex of a triangular flap. The TPF provides vascular perforators to the dermal plexus that supply the follicles; any incisions through the dermal plexus can compromise perfusion through this layer from the occipital, supraorbital, and contralateral STA vascular watersheds (**Fig. 6**).

Next, the remnant microtic cartilage is excised. This stage is performed by meticulous elevation of a very thin anteriorly based skin flap off the microtic cartilage, then coming under the cartilage mass and excising it. This flap frequently requires additional thinning when laying onto the pHDPE framework for optimal definition. The inferior portion of this flap typically has the lobule remnant attached to it initially. For improved soft tissue coverage, particularly with a malpositioned lobule, this flap may be amputated and used as a free skin graft. Amputation allows for improved ability to thin the skin; reserves that high-quality skin for use in the most aesthetically important areas (helical rim, scaphoid, antihelical flold (AHF) fossa triangularis) instead of the conchal bowl, which can tolerate darker skin if needed; and provides more flexibility in orientation. When removing the remnant microtic cartilage from the mastoid area, care must be taken not to injure a potentially anomalous course of the main trunk of the superficial temporal vascular pedicle that aberrantly courses under the cartilage. This possibility can be particularly relevant when removing excessive mastoid soft tissue down to the periosteal layer to create a deeper conchal bowl or in the setting of combined atresia-microtia cases in which the otologist requires subperiosteal elevation to expose the mastoid bone. Careful Doppler assessment of the vascular pedicle's trajectory

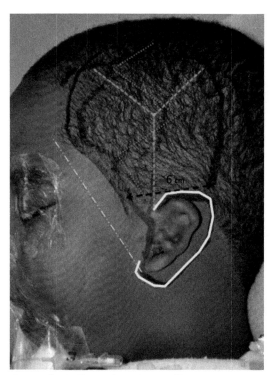

Fig. 6. Alternative scalp incisions. The Y or zigzag incision can be used for better access and visualization, but carry a higher risk for focal alopecia. (*From* Owen S, Wang T, Stephan S. Alloplastic reconstruction of the microtic ear. Operat Tech Otolaryngol Head Neck Surg 2017;28(2):99; with permission.)

immediately before surgery can help identify these anomalous cases.

Using the superior scalp incision, the temporoparietal area is widely undermined in a subcutaneous plane, with care taken not to violate either the TPF beneath or the hair follicles above. Once widely exposed, an inferiorly based TPF flap measuring approximately 10.5×13.0 cm is incised and elevated off the underlying deep temporal fascia (investing temporalis muscle) and the periosteum in the portion superior to the temporal line. Approximately one-third of the flap is superior to the temporal line, making it in practice a combination TPF extended by superficial parietal galeal aponeurosis. The base of the flap is kept wide (approximately 6 cm) to maximize inclusion of secondary vascular supply from the postauricular artery, early branches off the occipital artery, and the mastoid emissary vein. Although preserving every bit of the secondary vascular supply from this mastoid region is not always possible, every attempt is made to ensure the flap is as robust as possible with a redundant vascular supply (**Fig. 7**). Care is taken to preserve and include both the anterior and posterior branches

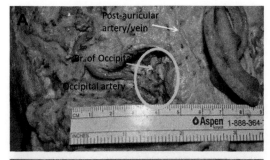

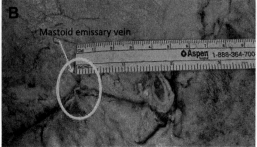

Fig. 7. Latex-injected cadaver dissections show the secondary vascular supply to the extended TPF flap from the mastoid region. If the base of the TPF flap is kept wide (~6 cm), several other vascular structures can be included in the mastoid area. (*A*) The postauricular artery and vein are located within 4 cm of an area posterior to the ear canal, as well as early branches (Br.) off the transverse portion of the occipital artery that course superiorly to the mastoid region. (*B*) Mastoid emissary vein is large, drains intracranial to the sigmoid sinus, and can often be incorporated if the flap base is kept wide.

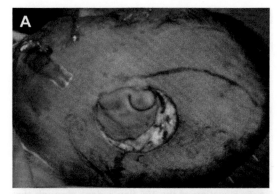

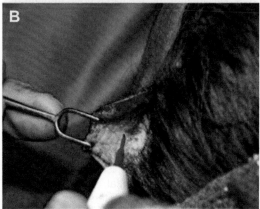

Fig. 8. (*A*) Postauricular incision made first and cartilage remnant removed leaving thin anteriorly based skin flap. (*B*) TPF flap elevation requires meticulous separation of subcutaneous fat away from superficial surface of TPF. (*From* Owen S, Wang T, Stephan S. Alloplastic reconstruction of the microtic ear. Operat Tech Otolaryngol Head Neck Surg 2017;28(2):99; with permission.)

of the superficial temporal artery, using electrocautery on a low setting to avoid thermal damage to the microvasculature. It is critical to include the loose areolar tissue on the deep surface of the TPF. This loose tissue will rest against the undersurface of the skin grafts and permit the skin to glide over the underlying structure, resisting soft tissue trauma and implant exposure. The flap is then reflected inferiorly through the superior portion of the posterior auricular incision (**Figs. 8** and **9**).

Next, the 2-piece pHDPE framework is sculpted and fused. The 2 separate implant pieces are placed in a 60-mL syringe of betadine, and placed under negative pressure to push antiseptic solution through the entire implant, not just coating the surface. The implant is tailored to the appropriate dimensions to match the contralateral ear. This process may be aided with the radiograph film template made from the contralateral ear. The pHDPE implant may be customized intraoperatively to appropriately mirror the patient's native anatomy. The implants are easily carved with a scalpel, and the 2 preformed components are then fused with high-heat ophthalmic cautery. The tragal extension and some portion of the lobule are routinely amputated in microtia cases; for auricular avulsion, anotia, or other complete ear reconstructions, the entire lobule can be preserved. The tragal portion is brittle and difficult to wrap with the TPF flap without blunting the bowl. The amputated pieces can be cut into many smaller fragments used to reinforce the implant. In particular, the union of the superior and inferior crura of the AHF to the helical rim requires reinforcement to avoid fracture and subluxation. Other modifications to the pHDPE framework can also be done, such as deepening of the conchal bowl and making the uniform helical rim irregular to provide a more natural appearance, as needed (**Figs. 10** and **11**).

Before placement of the implant, 2 flat suction drains are placed through the posterior mastoid

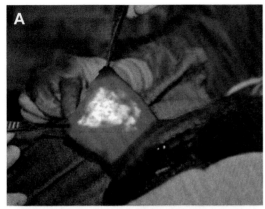

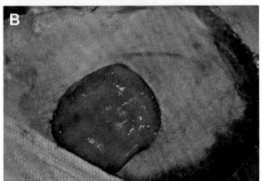

Fig. 9. (*A*) Vessels within thin TPF flap can be identified by transillumination. (*B*) TPF flap is delivered through a bipedicled scalp flap to the mastoid area. (*From* Owen S, Wang T, Stephan S. Alloplastic reconstruction of the microtic ear. Operat Tech Otolaryngol Head Neck Surg 2017;28(2):100; with permission.)

hair-bearing skin, with one deep to the pHDPE construct and the second in the posterior portion of the temporoparietal scalp donor site. The implant is then placed in the correct anatomic orientation, axis, and projection on the mastoid area and draped with the TPF flap. Confirmation of correct position is key at this stage because the implant cannot be adjusted easily after the flap is placed under negative pressure. The radiograph template created at the beginning of the procedure is used at this time to ensure correct placement. If projection needs to be altered, some excess of the implant can be shaved off the undersurface of the fused implant, or soldered on to it if needed at the inferior aspect, for example, for greater projection in the setting of a severely hypoplastic sloping temporal bone. The flap is oriented with the loose areolar layer facing away from the framework and then loosely secured to the mastoid fascia with a 5-0 polydioxanone suture. Strong fixation of the framework to the mastoid is avoided to maintain mobility of the ear, a feature needed to help absorb trauma and

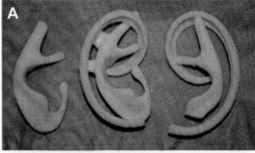

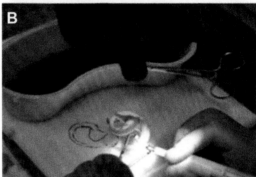

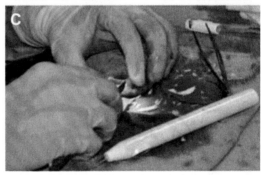

Fig. 10. (*A*) pHDPE implants come in 2 pieces to allow surgeons to adjust ear size as needed. There are slight variations by company on the shape of the preformed ear base, with some offering ready-made braces to buttress the helical rim (middle implant), as well as different arcs of curvature of the antihelical fold and the crura. (*B*) The 2 pieces are soldered together with ophthalmic cautery. (*C*) Further modifications using a scalpel can be done for optimization. (*From* Owen S, Wang T, Stephan S. Alloplastic reconstruction of the microtic ear. Operat Tech Otolaryngol Head Neck Surg 2017;28(2):100; with permission.)

resist framework fracture or soft tissue injury. If a native canal exists or a neocanal is being created during combined microtia-atresia surgery, then the implant position must be more fixated to the mastoid in order to avoid obstruction of the meatus by potential framework descent, even if it is subtle. A narrow strip of deep temporal fascia is raised and reflected through a window made in the base of the TPF serving as an inferiorly based

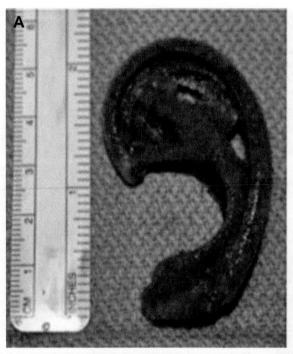
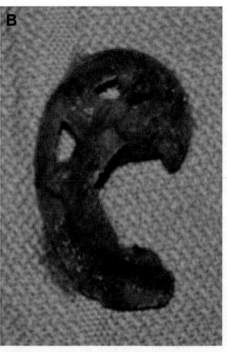

Fig. 11. Excess fragments of pHDPE such as shavings and amputated tragus/lobule component are used as material to reinforce the junctions between the 2 pieces. Finished product shows areas of reinforcement to prevent implant fractures. Helical root extension is amputated in cases with a canal or concurrent atresia surgery. Note that the implant is impregnated with iodine antiseptic solution. (*A*) Lateral surface of the implant; limited soldering or scalpel manipulation as possible (*B*) Medial (deep) surface of implant; primary area for soldering to reinforce. (*From* Owen S, Wang T, Stephan S. Alloplastic reconstruction of the microtic ear. Operat Tech Otolaryngol Head Neck Surg 2017;28(2):101; with permission.)

soft tissue sling. This fascial strip is wrapped around the inferior crus of the framework before covering the implant with the TPF flap.

The TPF flap is shrink-wrapped around the implant using negative pressure from the first drain. The second drain is for removal of any serous fluid from the TPF flap donor site (**Fig. 12**).

The anteriorly based skin flap is draped over the TPF, or amputated and positioned as a free skin graft. The lobule remnant typically requires inferior-posterior transposition, which is accomplished by sectioning it from the anteriorly based skin flap and transposing it based on a narrow anteriorly based pedicle (**Fig. 13**).

If the ipsilateral mastoid skin is not of sufficient surface area to cover the entire lateral surface of the new ear, a full-thickness skin graft is harvested from the contralateral postauricular sulcus. This graft provides the best color and texture match for the most aesthetically important parts of the reconstruction. A larger skin graft harvested from the inguinal region is typically required to cover the back of the ear. Care must be taken to adequately thin this graft, because it can be thick, even in children. Of note, the graft should also be

harvested as laterally as possible to prevent the inclusion of skin prone to grow pubic hair after puberty. Other donor site options include central lower abdominal skin, medial upper extremity, or supraclavicular fossa.

These harvested grafts are then combined to cover the new ear. The grafts will heal to resemble the original color and skin type from their donor regions. Because of this, the authors recommend that the ipsilateral auricular/mastoid skin be used on the lateral surface of the ear, with any gaps covered by the contralateral posterior auricular sulcus graft. The inguinal graft should be used primarily to resurface the new postauricular sulcus, because of its suboptimal color match. If possible, it is best to avoid inguinal skin anywhere on the helical rim, with the junction of the inguinal skin graft and the more favorable lateral surface grafts tucked behind on the medial surface of the auricle (**Fig. 14**).

For those reconstructions requiring a tragus, a small amount of the remnant ear cartilage is tailored into a tragal graft. This cartilage graft is then covered by the anteriormost portion of the anteriorly based preauricular skin flap. If this flap needs to be amputated for preferred lateral

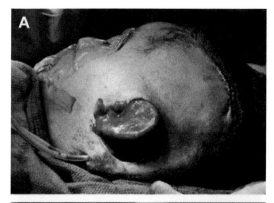

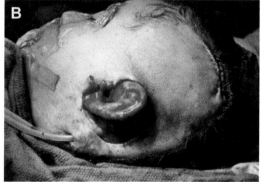

Fig. 12. (*A*) TPF flap draped over implant without suction. Anteriorly based skin flap has already been amputated. (*B*) Suction activated and flap shrink-wrapped around pHDPE framework. (*From* Owen S, Wang T, Stephan S. Alloplastic reconstruction of the microtic ear. Operat Tech Otolaryngol Head Neck Surg 2017;28(2):101; with permission.)

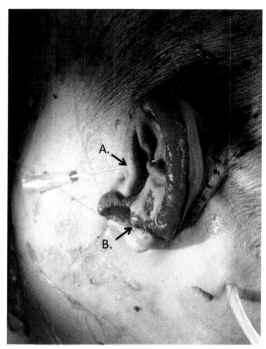

Fig. 13. Neotragus can be made by securing a cartilage graft tailored from previously resected microtic remnant to the anteriorly based mastoid skin flap (point A). The lobule can be partially split to set back inferiorly and hold the inferior portion of the TPF-wrapped implant like a sling (point B).

surface coverage, then a sufficient anterior portion is left attached to the preauricular skin to fold over a cartilage graft, braced temporarily with a needle, and secured using a 4-0 plain gut suture on a straight needle (see **Fig. 13**). Skin graft donor sites are closed, and skin grafts are attached to each other using absorbable gut suture. With the drains on suction, the auricle is coated with a thin layer of antibiotic ointment, gauze is tucked into concavities of the bowl, scaphoid, and fossa triangularis, and then the entire ear is covered in a custom silicone cast to prevent seroma, hematoma, or shearing trauma that may compromise skin graft viability during neovascularization. The silicone mold is secured to the scalp and skin with interrupted Prolene stitches. A Glasscock cup dressing is then applied to help prevent the weight of the silicone molding from pulling the auricle down. Pressure on the silicone mold should be avoided. Mastoid-style gauze pressure dressing is applied over the TPF donor site to prevent seroma formation.

Immediately following extubation, all suction drains are removed (**Figs. 15** and **16**).

AFTERCARE

The gauze pressure dressing is removed after 3 days and the parietal region inspected for seroma. The silicone mold is removed in clinic at 11 to 14 days. A new silicone mold is created in clinic for use behind the ear to maintain projection and avoid sulcus blunting against the forces of wound contracture. Patients wear this all night for 4 months. The silicone should not be worn during the day as the weight of the mold can contribute to inferior descent of the ear. Parents are asked to sleep with their children in the bed for the first few weeks to ensure that they do not roll onto the reconstructed ear. Aquaphor, Vaseline, or other moisturizing ointment is used until the wound edges and grafts cease to crust or scab.

DISCUSSION

Despite the popularity of autologous rib, pHDPE remains an excellent framework reconstructive option for ear surgeons. The primary advantages remain the avoidance of chest wall donor site

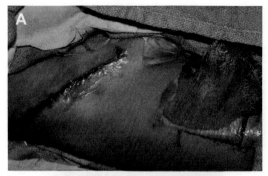

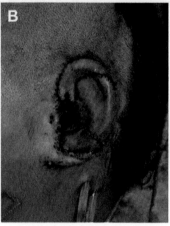

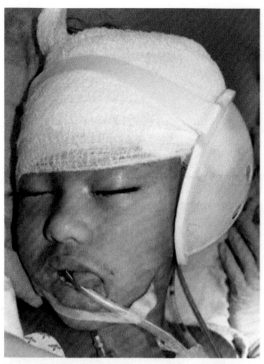

Fig. 15. Pink silicone mold covers the ear with a Glasscock cup dressing lifting mold slightly to support it. Gauze head wrap for pressure over TPF donor site. (*From* Owen S, Wang T, Stephan S. Alloplastic reconstruction of the microtic ear. Operat Tech Otolaryngol Head Neck Surg 2017;28(2):102; with permission.)

Fig. 14. (*A*) Inguinal donor full-thickness skin graft (FTSG) donor site closed primarily. Medial thigh split-thickness skin graft donor site used to line new canal during combined atresia surgery. (*B*) FTSG cover TPF flap. Lateral surface of ear covered by combination of previously amputated ipsilateral mastoid skin flap, contralateral postauricular FTSG, and remnant lobule. Inguinal skin only used for medial surface. Tragal reconstruction completed with small piece of remnant microtic cartilage. Patient also underwent canal atresiaplasty at the same time. (*From* Owen S, Wang T, Stephan S. Alloplastic reconstruction of the microtic ear. Operat Tech Otolaryngol Head Neck Surg 2017;28(2):102; with permission.)

morbidity, fewer stages, more consistent results, and the ability to perform an earlier repair. In most cases, this may be completed before the child starts school, minimizing the social impact of congenital deformity. Earlier repairs generally result in improved tissue healing and a more cosmetically appealing result.

Although it is easy to focus on choice of framework material as the key ingredient for success, outcomes depend mainly on soft tissue coverage.[4] The use of tissue expanders to allow complete coverage of the implant with preauricular tissue has been described as a viable option for soft tissue coverage. This technique has not been adopted by the authors because of the addition of an operative stage, potential tissue expander complications, the pain associated with expansion for children, and the fact that pHDPE often becomes exposed under a skin flap unless it is covered by an intervening fascia flap.

The ability to perform an entire repair in a single stage results in less recovery time, repetitive exposure to anesthesia, and care by patients and families. Preformed pHDPE implants allow less operative time carving rib frameworks, more predictability in the outcome, and an easier learning curve with respect to the framework design. However, microtia reconstruction in general requires meticulous attention to detail and superb soft tissue technique, regardless of what paradigm is used. As with any implantable material, there is concern for biofilm formation, infection, implant fracture, and extrusion. Although common in the early experience with pHDPE, modern techniques have significantly improved complication rates, which are now comparable with those of

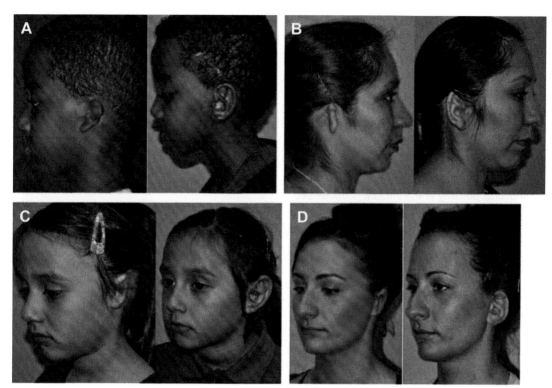

Fig. 16. (*A*, *B*) Primary reconstructions without canal atresia surgery. (*C*) Primary repair with combined atresia surgery. (*D*) Prior rib reconstruction revised with pHDPE approach. (*From* Owen S, Wang T, Stephan S. Alloplastic reconstruction of the microtic ear. Operat Tech Otolaryngol Head Neck Surg 2017;28(2):103; with permission.)

autologous rib techniques in experienced hands.[4,12] One study at a high-volume center examining long-term follow-up data elucidated no clear benefits to either autologous rib or pHDPE reconstruction.[11] Their conclusions were that pHDPE reconstructions had fewer operations and better size and contour match. Autologous rib advantages include better color match and decreased risk of extrusion.[11]

The senior author's experience implementing these changes over 28 years and their impact on rates of exposure, infection, and fractures is reflected in the notable trend toward reduced complication rate highlighted in **Table 1**. Several critical advancements in technique and materials that are responsible for this trend are discussed here.

RELIABILITY OF POROUS IMPLANTS

Early implant trials attempted the use of multiple different materials. Silicone was favored initially for its ability to mimic the flexibility of the native ear cartilage, but high exposure rates ultimately left it undesirable.[5] Polyethylene has a long history of biocompatibility, and the addition of micropores allows for vascular and soft tissue ingrowth. This advancement dramatically

improved resistance to infection and exposure.[19] Romo and colleagues[9] reported a 4% complication rate in 250 cases over an 11-year period, and Austrian surgeons with 78 cases report an extrusion rate of 2.6%.[20] The senior author's own experience from 2008 to 2013 detailed in **Table 1** is very similar. Other smaller-volume studies report complication rates between 0% and 12%.[10,11]

Table 1
Comparison of complication rates of porous high-density polyethylene ear reconstructions done by the senior author early in the series versus later in the series with implementation of several key technique advancements

	1993–1995	2008–2013
Procedures	25	487
Implant Fractures (%)	28	1.5–8.7
Implant Exposures (%)	44	4.3
Infections (%)	4	1.1

From Reinisch J. Ear reconstruction in young children. Facial Plast Surg 2015;31:601; with permission.

It follows that maintenance of the implant's porosity is important to the overall success, safety, and longevity of this technique. The junior author's preliminary investigations into this has yielded some interesting laboratory findings when analyzing electron microscopy images of pHDPE (Medpor samples) cut with a surgical scalpel as traditionally done, and compared with effects on porosity from soldering (as typically done for fusion of the 2-part implant), or sculpting the pHDPE with a drill using either a cutting bur or a diamond bur **Fig. 17**.

The overall porosity of the implant is decreased by any manipulation technique, but visual inspection shows only a modest decrease in porosity from baseline when pHDPE is cut with a scalpel, and only slightly worse than that when modified with a cutting bur using irrigation. However, all porosity seemed to be eliminated after soldering or diamond bur manipulation. Although the soldering is necessary to fuse the 2-piece implant together, minimizing the amount of soldering in the areas most prone to exposure is prudent. Clinical experience has shown the inferior portion of the helical rim where it fuses with the lobule

framework to be most vulnerable in this regard (especially in early recovery), because it is covered by the distal portion of the TPF flap and venous drainage must travel against gravity. Therefore, the safest technique to maintain porosity during framework modification is to use a scalpel and keep soldering to a minimum, and potentially only on the medial surfaces of the framework.

COVERAGE OF THE ENTIRE FRAMEWORK WITH THE VASCULARIZED TEMPOROPARIETAL FASCIA FLAP

In the early days of pHDPE ear reconstructions, only portions of the framework were covered with the TPF. The lower half of the implant was placed directly under the hairless mastoid skin, similar to how autologous rib reconstructions are now done. However, pHDPE requires more vascularized soft tissue coverage than autologous rib. In the early years, most exposures occurred at the sites covered under the mastoid skin inferior to the portion of the implant covered by the more vascularized fascia.[21] The dramatic decrease in exposure rate before and after this technical advancement is highlighted in **Table 1**.

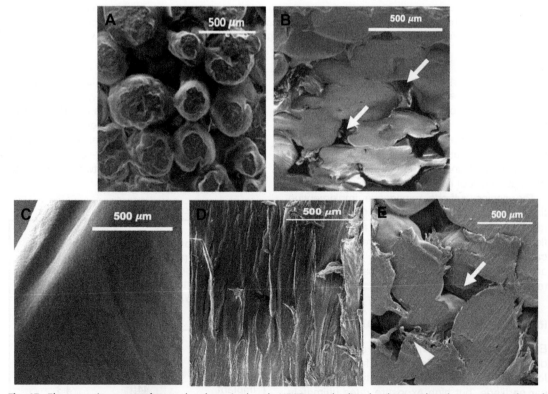

Fig. 17. Electron microscopy of control and manipulated pHDPE samples (Medpor). Note that the porosity is altered in all forms of manipulation, but minimally with scalpel cuts, and modestly with a cutter drill with irrigation. Significant loss of porosity seen with soldering or diamond drilling. (A) Normal pHDPE (control sample). (B) After scalpel cut. Arrows show some residual porosity. (C) After soldering with ophthalmic cautery. (D) After diamond drill with irrigation. (E) After cutter drill with irrigation. Arrow indicates maintained porosity, arrowhead shows implant spicules.

INCLUSION OF THE SUBGALEAL (AREOLAR) FASCIA WITH THE TEMPOROPARIETAL FASCIA FLAP

Traveling with the superficial temporal vessels is a sensory nerve making the TPF-covered ear implant sensate, a critical requirement for long-term viability and exposure prevention. However, if the overlying soft tissue is densely adherent to the implant, there is a much greater risk for exposure with normal auricular wear and tear. Over time the TPF undergoes tissue deposition and vascular ingrowth into the framework, which also makes it more adherent. Therefore, inclusion of the subgaleal loose areolar fascia with the harvest is important to avoid this problem. The loose areolar fascia is harvested off the superficial surface of the deep temporal fascia along with the flap. When transposed, this loose fascia now faces superficially and serves as a glide plane between the overlying skin grafts and the adherent TPF to resist soft tissue trauma and abrasion **(Fig. 18)**.[4]

REINFORCEMENT OF THE pHDPE FRAMEWORK

In the senior author's experience, early breakage of the implant, from rates as high as 25% in the first few years of practice, encouraged reinforcement along the superior portion of the implant.[21] These modifications reduced the fracture rate to 1.5% of ears without canals and 8.7% in ears with canals in a total of 487 patients operated on between 2008 and 2013 with average follow-up of 1.5 years. Weak areas of the framework may be structurally bolstered by soldering the extra implant pieces carved off from the lobule or unused tragal extension to the weakest points of fusion using high-temperature battery cautery. The most critical area to re-enforce is between the superior crus and lateral helical rim.

OCCIPITAL PARIETAL FLAP

Although the TPF is the ideal choice for primary reconstruction using a pHDPE implant, another

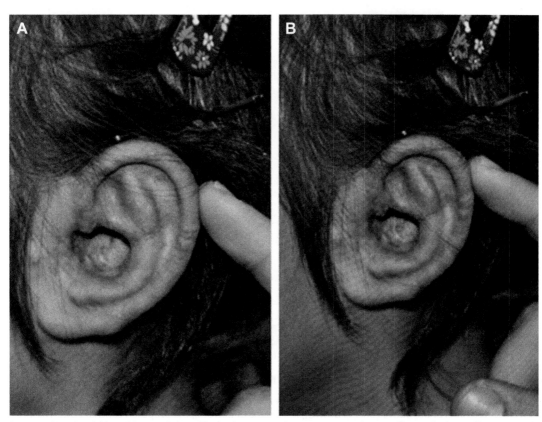

Fig. 18. Skin should be able to glide with the loose areolar tissue over the TPF flap, which is adherent to the pHDPE implant. Notice how the skin envelope glides over the framework between images (*A*) and (*B*). This ability allows some degree of protection from abrasion and blunt trauma. The TPF flap carries sensory fibers and the resultant ear skin is sensate to fine touch. (*From* Owen S, Wang T, Stephan S. Alloplastic reconstruction of the microtic ear. Operat Tech Otolaryngol Head Neck Surg 2017;28(2):104; with permission.)

regional flap is available if needed:– the occipital parietal (OCP) flap based on the axial supply of the occipital artery and vein. Anatomically, the OCP flap is the superficial occipito-parietal fascia that is the posterior continuation of the TPF, all part of the epicranial aponeurosis (or galea aponeurotica). This flap can be used in the setting of revision after a failed TPF-based reconstruction using a pHDPE implant, serving as a plan B if problems occur. There are other scenarios in which an OCP flap is necessary: if the superficial temporal vessels or the TPF are compromised from prior scarring, burn, or surgery; when previously banked rib cartilage over the main STA bifurcation creates undue risk for vascular compromise or excessive flap thickness; if there is a malpositioned bone-anchored abutment for hearing appliances or prosthesis. The OCP flap is comparable with the TPF in thickness and pliability, also has a paired

sensory nerve with it, and typically yields similar aesthetic results to the TPF. However, the OCP flap harvest can be more challenging because it is further away from the mastoid region and requires a longer flap with more dissection below the nuchal line to allow for rotation and transposition (**Fig. 19**).

HARVEST OF A WIDE-BASED TEMPOROPARIETAL FASCIA FLAP

The TPF flap shows variability of both arterial and venous flow in up to 37% of patients.[22] The authors recommend the use of Doppler ultrasonography intraoperatively to confirm arterial supply patterns, and keeping as wide a base to the TPF flap as possible to improve venous and lymphatic outflow and inclusion of potential contributions from the posterior auricular, emissary, and

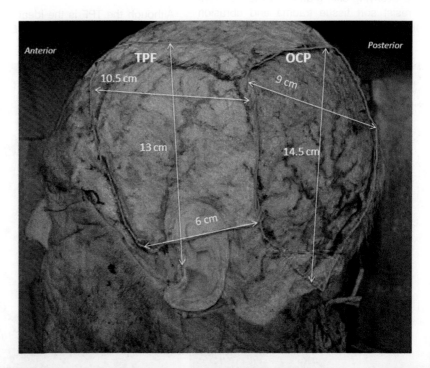

TPF Flap	Width (cm)	Length (cm) from canal	OCP Flap	Width (cm)	Length (cm) from 90° kink
Min. size	8.5 (±0.47)	11.05 (±0.44)	Min. size	8.6 (±0.81)	13.05 (±0.55)
Recommend	**10.5**	**12.5–13**	**Recommend**	**9**	**14–14.5**

Fig. 19. Latex-injected cadaver dissections show recommended dimensions of a TPF flap and an OCP flap. Vertical height for a TPF starts at the native conchal bowl or, in the case of microtia, the proposed conchal bowl. The TPF is transposed by flipping it down to the ear area like turning a page in a book. The OCP flap vertical height measurement begins approximately 1 cm below the nuchal line (*green dashed line*) where the main occipital vessels abruptly make a right-angle turn superiorly and penetrate the deep cervical fascia investing the trapezius muscle. The OCP flap is relocated to the ear area in a similar way as the TPF flip maneuver but also requires some rotation with the axis of pivot located at the nuchal line.

occipital vessels (see **Fig. 7**). Narrowing of the TPF pedicle base to include exclusively the main trunk of the superficial temporal vessels can be tempting intraoperatively, because the flap is much more mobile and can drape more easily over the implant with less potential folding in the sulcus area. However, this narrowing comes at the cost of the secondary vascularity provided from the mastoid region, which in our estimation is important to maintain.

Cadaveric studies using latex injection of the galeal vasculature by these authors helped to corroborate the clinical experience on recommended flap dimensions used over the years (see **Fig. 19**). A pHDPE implant tailored to normative adult dimensions (implant sized to 53 × 31 mm to accommodate additions of soft tissue envelope and lobule generating a 60 × 33 mm adult ear of normative dimensions)[18] is covered by a raised TPF flap placed under negative pressure. The flaps were made smaller and smaller until minimum dimensions required to maintain a negative pressure seal were determined. This minimum size for both TPF and OCP flaps helped guide the recommendations listed in the table. These investigations also showed what portions of the TPF flap cover the different subunits of the auricular framework (**Figs. 20** and **21**). The inferior helical rim, midhelical rim, and antitragus are the locations that can have the highest risk for exposure over the long term. Verifying excellent vascularity of the flap along these key locations and maintaining the secondary blood supply from the mastoid region can help prevent future problems.

FUTURE DEVELOPMENTS

Several exciting areas of innovation are emerging in alloplast-based auricular reconstruction. Customized implants made from computed tomography or MRI data of the contralateral ear offer the prospect of an identical match and have already been used in the setting of unilateral microtia. What remains to be seen is whether the significant increase in cost of creating this three-dimensional (3D) printed replica is balanced by a clearly demonstrable aesthetic improvement. Similar to rib reconstruction, the difference between a less than average result and an excellent outcome often depends not on the framework but on the soft tissue that is covering it. One advantage of the 3D customized implant is that it is a single structure not requiring fusion, which saves operative time and theoretically is stronger than the fused 2-piece implant.

Alloplast microtia frameworks may also have a role in stem cell–based auricular reconstruction. One of the great challenges facing rib microtia surgeons is the many inflammatory mediators and contractile forces that surround the autologous rib framework through the multitude of stages involved

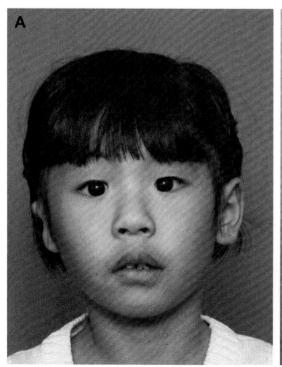
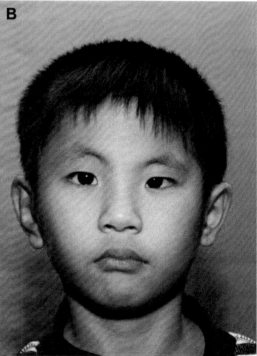

Fig. 20. Single stage, outpatient pHDPE ear reconstruction. (*A*) Preoperative. (*B*) One year postoperative.

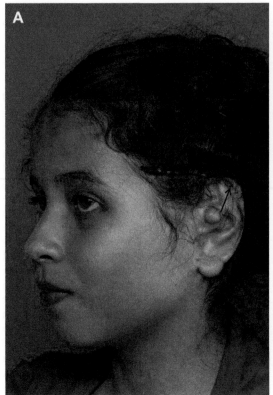 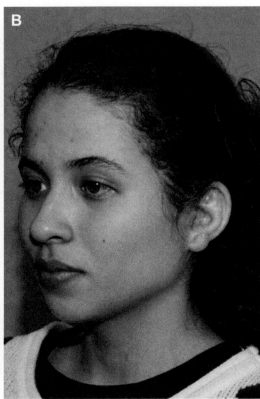

Fig. 21. Referral case with implant exposure following scalp tissue expander and placement of the implant under the expanded skin only. (*A*) Pre-op with arrow showing site of exposure at the helical rim. The STA was injured during the original placement of the expander. (*B*) Salvage done using occipital galeal flap (OCP) and replacement of the implant. Seen 3 years after OCP flap over new implant.

over time. These factors influence how much resorption may occur, leading to loss of detail, projection, and architecture. For those scientists trialing tissue-engineered auricular frameworks in animal models, these inflammatory and contractile forces often decimate the architecture and strength of the cartilage. pHDPE could be used as the primary stage, covering it with TPF and skin grafts in the standard fashion, while the chondrocytes harvested from the auricular remnant are cultured and prepared on scaffolds as many researchers have tried. The difference is that this bioengineered autologous cartilage framework could be swapped with the pHDPE implant in a second stage into a ready-made precontracted soft tissue envelope. The alloplast plays its part in bearing the brunt of soft tissue contracture and then makes way for an autologous, flexible framework to be inserted.

SUMMARY

The use of pHDPE as an alloplast in microtia reconstruction offers an excellent framework for pediatric reconstructive surgeons. Advantages include earlier reconstruction, fewer procedures,

avoidance of donor site morbidity, shorter learning curve, and improved size and contour match. Results ultimately depend on soft tissue envelope, and choice of technique is best decided according to surgeon expertise and patient preference.

REFERENCES

1. Im DD, Paskhover B, Staffenberg DA, et al. Current management of microtia—a national survey. Aesthetic Plast Surg 2013;37:402–8.
2. Owen S, Wang T, Stephan S. Alloplastic reconstruction of the microtic ear. Operat Tech Otolaryngol Head Neck Surg 2017;28(2):97–104.
3. Reinisch JF. Ear reconstruction with porous polyethylene implant—an 8 year surgical experience. Colorado Springs (CO): American Association of Plastic Surgeons; 1999.
4. Reinisch JF, Lewin S. Ear reconstruction using a porous polyethylene framework and temporoparietal fascia flap. Facial Plast Surg 2009;25(3):181–9.
5. Cronin TD. Use of a Silastic frame for total and subtotal reconstruction of the external ear: preliminary report. Plast Reconstr Surg 1966;37:399–405.

6. Berghaus A. Porecon implant and fan flap: a concept for reconstruction of the auricle. Facial Plast Surg 1988;133(1):111–20.

7. Wellisz T. Clinical experience with the Medpor porous polyethylene implant. Aesthetic Plast Surg 1993;17(4):339–44.

8. Spector M, Harmon SL, Kreutner A. Characteristics of tissue growth into Proplast and porous polyethylene implants in bone. J Biomed Mater Res 1979; 13(5):677–92.

9. Romo T 3rd, Morris LG, Reitzen SD, et al. Reconstruction of congenital microtia-atresia: outcomes with the Medpor/bone-anchored hearing aid–approach. Ann Plast Surg 2009;62(4):384–9.

10. Yang SL, Zheng JH, Ding Z, et al. Combined fascial flap and expanded skin flap for enveloping Medpor framework in microtia reconstruction. Aesthetic Plast Surg 2009;33(4):518–22.

11. Constantine KK, Gilmore J, Lee K, et al. Comparison of microtia reconstruction outcomes using rib cartilage vs porous polyethylene implant. JAMA Facial Plast Surg 2014;16(4):240–4.

12. Long X, Yu N, Huang J, et al. Complication rate of autologous cartilage microtia reconstruction: a systematic review. Plast Reconstr Surg Glob Open 2013;1(7):e57.

13. Brent B. The pediatrician's role in caring for patients with congenital microtia and atresia. Pediatr Ann 1999;28:374–83.

14. Bradbury ET, Hewison J, Timmons MJ. Psychological and social outcome of prominent ear correction in children. Br J Plast Surg 1992;45:97–100.

15. Jiamei D, Jiake C, Hongxing Z, et al. An investigation of psychological profiles and risk factors in congenital microtia patients. J Plast Reconstr Aesthet Surg 2008;61(Suppl 1):S37–43.

16. Lee TS, Lim SY, Pyon JK, et al. Secondary revisions due to unfavourable results after microtia reconstruction. J Plast Reconstr Aesthet Surg 2010;63(6):940–6.

17. Park C, Mun HY. Use of an expanded temporoparietal fascial flap technique for total auricular reconstruction. Plast Reconstr Surg 2006;118(2):374–82.

18. Sforza C, Grandi G, Binelli M, et al. Age- and sex-related changes in the normal human ear. Forensic Sci Int 2009;187(1–3):110.e1-7.

19. Berghaus A, Axhausen M, Handrock M. Porous synthetic material in external ear reconstruction. Laryngol Rhinol Otol (Stuttg) 1983;62:320–7 [in German].

20. Kludt NA, Vu H. Auricular reconstruction with prolonged tissue expansion and porous polyethylene implants. Ann Plast Surg 2014;72(Suppl 1):S14–7.

21. Reinisch J. Ear reconstruction in young children. Facial Plast Surg 2015;31(6):600–3.

22. Park C, Lew DH, Yoo WM. An analysis of 123 temporoparietal fascial flaps: anatomic and clinical considerations in total auricular reconstruction. Plast Reconstr Surg 1999;104(5):1295–306.

Atresiaplasty in Congenital Aural Atresia
What the Facial Plastic Surgeon Needs to Know

Douglas S. Ruhl, MD, MSPH, Bradley W. Kesser, MD*

KEYWORDS

- Atresia • Microtia • Otologist • Congenital aural atresia • Atresiaplasty • Canalplasty
- Atresia surgery • Conductive hearing loss

KEY POINTS

- Evaluation of hearing early in life is essential in patients with congenital aural atresia so options for early auditory habilitation can be presented to the family.
- Bone conduction hearing devices are a necessity in children with bilateral microtia/atresia to support normal speech and language development.
- Microtia surgery with rib grafting should precede canalplasty; however, canalplasty should precede microtia repair when the Medpor or SuPor implant is used.
- Surgeons must consider the possibility of an aberrant or superficial facial nerve in these patients.
- It is imperative that the reconstructive surgeon and the otologist work together to coordinate care.

INTRODUCTION

Patients with congenital aural atresia (CAA) present with a spectrum of severity that ranges from ear canal stenosis to complete absence of the external auditory canal. This rarely occurs in isolation, but is more commonly associated with microtia or other craniofacial dysplasias (see later). The middle ear and ossicles are affected to varying degrees.[1] It has been estimated that CAA occurs in 1 out of 10,000 to 20,000 births.[2] Males are more commonly affected than females, and atresia affects the right ear more frequently than the left ear. Unilateral atresia is much more common than bilateral atresia (3- to 7-fold difference).[1,3] Approximately 10% of patients with CAA have an associated syndrome including Treacher Collins, Goldenhar, hemifacial microsomia, branchio-oto-renal syndrome, de Grouchy, and Crouzon, so a careful physical examination is important during the initial visit.[3]

Patients with microtia and atresia may face multiple surgeries to correct the malformation. Ideally, children should be evaluated at a multidisciplinary center shortly after birth. These children require the services of an audiologist, otologist, reconstructive surgeon, speech therapist, and possibly a developmental pediatrician. The parents and child face many difficult decisions. How will they address the hearing problem? Should they correct the microtia? Should the child have canalplasty surgery? When should one order the computed tomography (CT) scan to evaluate for canal surgery? Who should do these surgeries, and at what age?

Disclosure Statement: The authors have nothing to disclose.
Department of Otolaryngology–Head and Neck Surgery, University of Virginia School of Medicine, PO Box 800713, Charlottesville, VA 22908, USA
* Corresponding author.
E-mail address: bwk2n@virginia.edu

Facial Plast Surg Clin N Am 26 (2018) 87–96
https://doi.org/10.1016/j.fsc.2017.09.005
1064-7406/18/© 2017 Elsevier Inc. All rights reserved.

This article discusses several important aspects of atresia surgery that the reconstructive surgeon should be aware of to ensure that these patients have comprehensive care with optimal outcomes.

ASSESSING HEARING

When a child is diagnosed with microtia/atresia, usually in the newborn nursery, the hearing should be assessed as early as possible with air and bone conduction auditory brainstem response testing. Auditory brainstem response testing is mandatory in the postnatal period to determine hearing thresholds in both ears.[4] Typically, the atretic ear has a moderate to severe conductive hearing loss with air conduction thresholds in the 50- to 65-dB hearing level range and normal bone conduction thresholds (0- to 10-dB hearing level). In patients with unilateral microtia/atresia, the hearing status of the contralateral (normal) ear is equally, if not more important. It should not be assumed that the hearing is normal in the nonatretic ear just because the external ear looks normal. Air conduction auditory brainstem response testing should be performed in the contralateral, normal ear to verify normal hearing.

When the child is older, behavioral audiometry with air and bone conduction testing should be done to continue to monitor hearing status and cochlear integrity. Children between ages 1 and 3 can be tested behaviorally with visual reinforced audiometry and those ages 3 to 6 with conditioned play audiometry.[3] Testing is generally recommended every 3 to 6 months for the first 2 years of life, and if the hearing is stable, every 6 to 12 months thereafter.

HEARING HABILITATION

Based on audiometric testing results, options are presented to the family for hearing habilitation. Use of a soft or hardband bone conducting hearing device is a necessity for normal speech and language development in children with bilateral CAA. In children with unilateral CAA, the data are not as convincing about the benefits of a bone conducting device. Although normal hearing in one ear is sufficient for normal speech and language development, the long-term effects of aiding versus not aiding the atretic ear (with a bone conducting device) are unknown. Parents should never be discouraged from having their child with unilateral CAA use a bone conductor, but the necessity or the benefits of a bone conductor in a child with unilateral CAA remains under investigation.[5]

In children with bilateral CAA, the bone conducting device should be fit as early as possible and worn until the child is at an age where additional options (eg, canal surgery; osseointegrated bone conducting device, such as the BAHA system [Cochlear Americas, Englewood, CO] or Ponto [Oticon Corp, Somerset, NJ]) are available. During the interim, however, it is important to ensure that adequate auditory input is presented during the child's critical language development period between the ages of 0 and approximately 8.

Older children have several options regarding hearing habilitation. For children with unilateral CAA, parents may elect to do nothing and simply monitor the hearing and speech and language development, providing benefits in the classroom, such as preferential seating, a frequency modulated (FM) system, or other resources through an individualized educational plan (IEP).[5] Implantable, osseointegrated bone conducting devices are an excellent option for patients with bilateral CAA, if the family does not wish to pursue canalplasty, or for patients who are poor candidates for surgery.[6] The hearing outcomes of these devices are consistently excellent, often equivalent or better than the audiometric results gained from canalplasty.[6–9] However, these devices have some drawbacks. The Food and Drug Administration prohibits implanting patients less than 5 years old. These devices do not support good sound localization. Some patients find the device cumbersome, and they can have wound care issues, such as inflammation, granulation, moisture at the site, or skin overgrowth. These skin issues could be a significant problem for the reconstructive surgeon if the device is placed too close to the surgical field for the auricular reconstruction. Communication between otologist and reconstructive surgeon is critical so that the osseointegrated bone conducting device is placed in a favorable position for auricular reconstruction.

Atresia surgery, when performed properly and in the appropriate patient, can achieve outstanding hearing results. Even if hearing results decline over time, having an external auditory canal can allow the patient to wear a traditional in-the-ear hearing aid, which may bring the hearing into the normal range.[8]

Parents hunger for solid, reliable information about microtia/atresia, and early consultation with an experienced reconstructive surgeon and otologist starts their journey off on the right track even if nothing, other than monitoring the hearing, needs to be done in the 0- to 4-year-old child's life. After the early auditory needs have been met, the child's candidacy for auricular and/or atresia surgery is undertaken around the age of 4 to 5.

Microtia reconstruction with autologous rib grafting generally occurs around age 5 to 6, when the costal cartilage has reached a size adequate for harvesting and carving into the auricle. Reconstruction with a porous polyethylene implant (Medpor [Stryker Corp, Kalamazoo, MI] or SuPor [Poriferous, LLC, Newnan, GA]) is possible at the age of 3, but canalplasty is not recommended until the child is older, around the age of 6 to 7.

Atresia surgery is not recommended until the child is 6 to 7 for several reasons. The older child with CAA understands the purpose and goals of the operation and is more cooperative in the office with the delicate packing removal and debridement of the ear to ensure a good result. Second, the older child has a greater chance of having outgrown any eustachian tube issues that could cause fluid in the middle ear or otitis media with effusion after surgery. Third, the older child may be less likely to experience postoperative canal stenosis because new bone growth and meatal stenosis are more common in younger children. Fourth, it is important to establish accurate preoperative and postoperative behavioral auditory (air and bone conduction) thresholds. Younger children are not as reliable and may not be able to participate or cooperate for comprehensive behavioral audiometry. Finally, to assess candidacy for atresia surgery, the otologic surgeon needs a high-resolution CT scan. There is no reason to subject the younger, smaller child to the radiation dose of a CT scan and its attendant risks at the age of 2 or 3 when surgery is not performed until 6 to 7.

NONSURGICAL REPAIR

The family should be presented the option of a prosthetic ear. Prosthetic specialists are skilled in skin color match, placement, and overall appearance. The prosthetic ear is affixed to the skin with medical tape or with osseointegrated implants (eg, Vistafix, Cochlear Americas). The prosthetic specialist can build the prosthetic ear (or make a meatus) around the reconstructed ear canal after atresia surgery if the family wishes to pursue atresia repair.

SURGICAL REPAIR
Who Should Perform Microtia/Atresia Surgery?

Like any surgery, microtia and atresia reconstruction should be performed by experienced surgeons who treat a large number of these patients. The first attempt at cosmetic reconstruction is the best attempt so an experienced surgeon should perform the operation. Plastic surgeons

and facial plastic surgeons are the primary reconstructive specialists for repairing microtia. If the first set of surgeries fails to achieve an acceptable result, there is little chance that supplemental operations will greatly improve the appearance of the ear.[4] Polyethylene implants (eg, Medpor or SuPor) are more forgiving in this regard, and can be potentially used after failed rib graft. The family must be informed of the potential risks of extrusion, fracture of the framework, and exposure.

Need for Microtia Reconstruction

Microtia reconstruction is often considered for cosmetic and functional benefits (ie, to facilitate wearing glasses or behind-the-ear hearing aids). Not every patient with congenital microtia benefits from auricular reconstruction. For example, a patient with grade I microtia (small ear with mostly normal anatomy) almost never needs microtia surgery. However, a patient with grade III microtia (the most common form characterized by a small peanut-like vestige) is almost always a candidate for auricular reconstruction (**Fig. 1**). It may be difficult to improve on a grade II microtia (partially developed auricle with tragus present), and the patient may instead elect to proceed directly to atresia repair (**Fig. 2**).[4] Ultimately, it is up to the

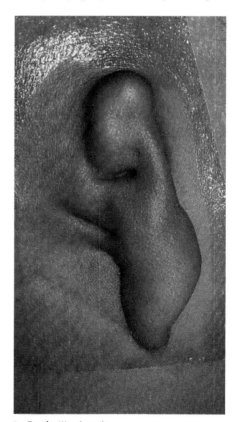

Fig. 1. Grade III microtia.

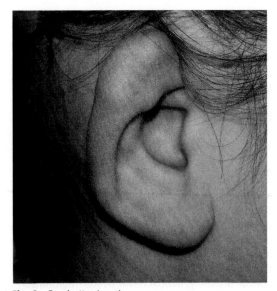

Fig. 2. Grade II microtia.

Table 1
Jahrsdoerfer grading system of candidacy for surgery of congenital aural atresia

Parameter	Points
Stapes present	2
Oval window open	1
Middle ear space	1
Facial nerve normal	1
Malleus-incus complex present	1
Mastoid well pneumatized	1
Incus-stapes connection	1
Round window normal	1
Appearance of external ear	1
Total points available	10

Rating	Type of Candidate
10	Excellent
9	Very good
8	Good
7	Fair
6	Marginal
≤5	Poor

From Jahrsdoerfer RA, Yeakley JW, Aguilar EA, et al. Grading system for the selection of patients with congenital aural atresia. Am J Otol 1992;13:7; with permission.

patient and family to decide if they wish to pursue auricular reconstruction and by which method (prosthesis vs rib graft vs Medpor). This decision is critical, because it has implications for atresia surgery, as discussed later.

Surgical Candidacy for Atresia Repair

Successful atresiaplasty aims to give the patient a clean, dry, epithelialized ear canal with a widely patent meatus and improved hearing. When evaluating patients for canalplasty surgery, it is incumbent on the otologist to ensure that surgery is performed safely and that the patient has a good chance of hearing improvement. Several classification systems can help predict postoperative hearing outcomes. The Jahrsdoerfer score is the most commonly used system to assess surgical candidacy and prognosticate hearing outcomes (**Table 1**).[10] This grading system assesses nine anatomic components from the CT scan and physical examination. Higher scores are associated with better postoperative hearing outcomes. Patients with a Jahrsdoerfer score of seven or higher have significantly better hearing outcomes compared with those with a score of six or lower.[10,11]

Although classification systems to evaluate surgical candidacy for CAA are useful, they rely on subjective interpretation of many variables. Middle ear aeration is regarded as the most important factor in determining postoperative success.[11,12] Also, better preoperative hearing strongly predicts better postoperative hearing and often correlates with ear anatomy.[13]

The auricular reconstructive surgeon should know that, when followed long term, some patients experience decline in hearing, and they may pursue revision canal surgery. Other long-term issues include canal stenosis from scar tissue or new bone growth, loss of the skin graft with mucosalization of the canal and a "wet" ear, and ossicular refixation or lateralization of the new tympanic membrane with hearing loss and widening of the air bone gap.[14–16] It is unclear if patients with atresia have problems with their eustachian tube that may predispose them to middle ear dysfunction. In our experience, younger patients are more likely to have bony regrowth compared with adults who have primary atresia surgery. Patients must also be counseled that they need routine cleaning of canal debris once or twice per year.

Surgeons should be cautious and avoid performing canalplasty in certain situations. Surgery should not be performed if an aberrant facial nerve travels across the area where the external auditory canal should be or blocks access to the oval window with an absent stapes bone. A low tegmen and/or poorly pneumatized mastoid and/or constricted middle ear space may prevent access to the atretic plate/ossicles or result in poor hearing outcomes. Also, surgery should be avoided if the middle ear is opacified on the CT scan.

Who Goes First: Reconstructive Surgeon or Otologist?

The timing of the microtia and atresia procedures should be in the patient's best interest to ensure the finest possible cosmetic appearance. The order of the surgeries is dependent on the family's decision for microtia repair: autologous rib graft versus Medpor/SuPor reconstruction (for the remainder of the article, we simply refer to Medpor with the understanding that the SuPor implant is also used). Atresia surgery can also be performed without auricular reconstruction or with a prosthetic ear.

Rib graft microtia repair

Classically, microtia repair has been performed in a three- or four-stage procedure with autologous rib cartilage.[1,17,18] These operations include (1) cartilage harvest from the 9th and 10th ribs and implantation of the sculpted framework in a subcutaneous pocket, (2) transposition of the external ear remnant to become the new lobule, (3) elevation of the auricle with skin grafting, and (4) tragal reconstruction. Several modifications have been proposed that combine stages to decrease the number of surgeries.[18–21] Regardless, we recommend performing atresia repair at a minimum (there is no maximum time limit) of 3 to 6 months after the last stage of microtia repair. Occasionally, the tragal reconstruction is performed last, and atresia surgery is done between the ear elevation and tragal reconstruction. Atresia surgery can also be performed before the ear has been elevated, between stages 2 and 3 mentioned previously.

When rib grafting is used for microtia repair, the cosmetic surgeries should precede atresia repair. This gives the reconstructive surgeon the opportunity to operate in pristine tissue with excellent blood supply and without scar. Although the new bony external auditory canal can only be placed in one location (generally just inferior to the root of the zygoma and just posterior to the glenoid fossa), the reconstructed auricle can be carefully undermined and moved slightly to align the lateral meatus with the bony canal (**Fig. 3**).

The osseointegrated bone conducting device should also be performed after the rib graft microtia repair, but an experienced otologist can place the device far enough posteriorly and away so as not to interfere with the area for the rib graft. The device's processor must also not touch the

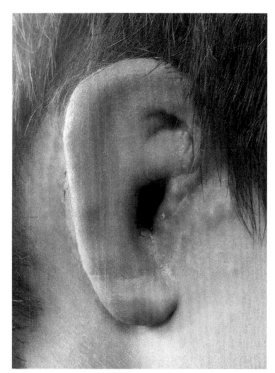

Fig. 3. Atresia surgery after rib graft reconstruction. Bony canal aligns with soft tissue meatus.

reconstructed auricle lest the patient have annoying feedback.

Medpor/SuPor microtia repair

Use of Medpor porous polyethylene framework for microtia reconstruction has increased in popularity. This approach offers fewer surgeries for the patient and has excellent cosmetic outcomes when performed in experienced hands. A recent comparison among atresiaplasty with Medpor, atresiaplasty with rib graft, and atresiaplasty alone showed similar hearing results in all groups; interestingly, the Medpor group had less meatal stenosis.[22]

When Medpor microtia reconstruction is to be performed, it is important that the atresia surgery be performed first (**Fig. 4**). Atresia surgery before Medpor reconstruction helps guide the reconstructive surgeon where to place the auricle. More importantly, however, performing the atresia surgery after the Medpor implant is placed needlessly puts the implant at risk of being exposed. If exposed during the atresia operation, skin does not heal over the polyethylene implant, and the child needs another operation for coverage of the exposed area. Additionally, the atresia operation could put the vascular pedicle of the temporoparietal fascia flap (the delicate flap that covers the implant) at risk. Finally, the stiffer Medpor

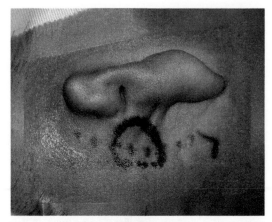

Fig. 4. Atresia surgery is performed before Medpor implant surgery. Note the location of the postauricular incision and how the future meatus is incorporated into the postauricular incision.

auricle cannot be easily moved after reconstruction to align the meatus to the bony canal, so atresiaplasty must be first in this situation (**Fig. 5**).

For the osseointegrated bone conducting device, the Medpor reconstruction should again go first so the titanium abutment/implant is not in the way of the polyethylene implant, and the surgery does not jeopardize the vascular supply of

the temporoparietal fascia flap. Some reconstructive surgeons are learning to do the osseointegrated implant surgery, and these two operations can be done at the same time.

HEARING OUTCOMES

Studies of postoperative hearing outcomes in patients undergoing atresia repair suffer from a lack of long-term follow-up. In the early postoperative period, hearing gains are good, with many, if not most, patients achieving pure tone averages and speech reception thresholds in the normal or near-normal range.[3,13–16] Hearing outcomes are clearly related to anatomy: the more well-formed the middle ear structures and anatomy (as documented by the Jahrsdoerfer grading scale), the better the hearing outcomes.[10–12,23]

Hearing results are no different when comparing outcomes in patients undergoing atresia surgery after rib graft microtia repair with patients undergoing atresia surgery before Medpor repair.[22]

Few studies have looked at long-term hearing outcomes, but these studies do show some decline in hearing (air conduction) thresholds over time in a subset of patients, approximately 20% to 30%.[14,15] Theories behind this decline include new bone formation during puberty that

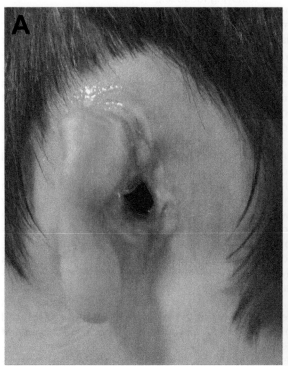
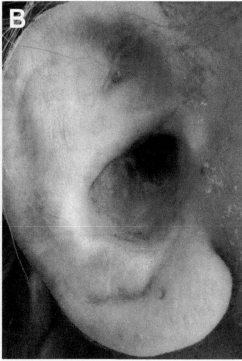

Fig. 5. Location of the meatus and canal after canalplasty surgery before (*A*) and after (*B*) Medpor reconstructive surgery.

refixes the ossicles, scar tissue that refixes the os-sicles, and lateralization of the tympanic membrane. Revision surgery for hearing loss alone is often successful in restoring hearing, but no long-term studies have examined hearing stability after revision surgery.[24]

Compared with atresia surgery, placement of an osseointegrated bone conducting hearing device results in better hearing and more reliable hearing improvement with less variability in hearing outcomes.[6–8] For children with unilateral atresia, however, it is unclear whether these osseointegrated bone conduction devices address or improve the two fundamental problems associated with unilateral hearing loss: sound localization and hearing in background noise. Studies have shown improvement of hearing in background noise after atresia repair,[25–27] and, after atresia surgery, patients located sound better in background noise as compared with preoperative values.[27,28]

A final consideration is observation without surgery or direct amplification. Children with unilateral atresia did not fail a grade in elementary school and did better than their peers with unilateral sensorineural hearing loss.[5] These children did use resources (IEPs, 504[c] plans, FM systems), but few (12%) used any type of amplification.[5]

Much like the decision for microtia repair, the decision to observe and use educational resources, such as an FM system or IEP, versus placing a bone conducting hearing device versus atresia surgery for the child with CAA is an individualized, family decision. The decision is best made when all options are presented in a clear and objective fashion. Physicians evaluating and managing children with microtia/atresia should be aware of the risks and benefits of each of these options. The otologic or pediatric otolaryngologic surgeon should be in contact with the microtia reconstructive surgeon to ensure optimal cosmetic and functional results.

IMPORTANT CONSIDERATIONS
The Presence of Cholesteatoma

If a family wishes to have their child evaluated for canalplasty, a fine-cut CT scan of the temporal bones should be obtained when the patient is around 5 years old. Patients with congenital aural stenosis are also at a small, but increased risk of harboring an ear canal cholesteatoma, which should be readily apparent on the imaging by this age. It has been estimated that up to 20% of patients with congenital aural stenosis (as defined by a canal diameter of 2 mm or less) may have cholesteatoma.[29]

Any patient with microtia/atresia who has concomitant cholesteatoma should have the canal surgery first. In this situation, eradication of the disease should take precedent over auricular reconstruction.[4,29]

The Conchal Bowl and Tragus

It is imperative that the rib graft reconstructive surgeon build a conchal bowl within the overall framework of the auricle. This depression must coincide with proper placement of tragal cartilage and bony canal to give the best chance of a normal-appearing auricle.[4] An important point: the bony canal cannot be moved; thus, the conchal bowl (and future site of the meatus) of the rib graft reconstruction must closely approximate where the bony canal will be. Another important point: the bony canal in children undergoing atresia repair is centered at the epitympanum, not meso-tympanum, so the placement of the conchal bowl and ultimately the entire framework should cheat 1 to 2 cm superiorly if the child will undergo atresia surgery for optimal alignment between the meatus (conchal bowl) and future site of the bony canal.

The otologist may use the conchal skin as a skin flap (anteriorly based hinged at the base of the tragus; **Fig. 6**) to line the anterior lateral canal

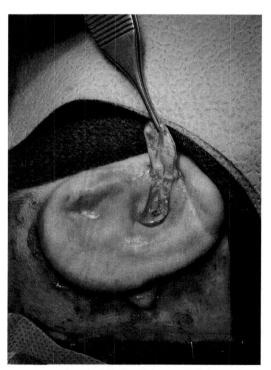

Fig. 6. Anteriorly based conchal skin flap to be directed medially through the newly created meatus to serve as the anterolateral canal skin.

wall. It is therefore important that this conchal skin be aligned properly to the future site of the bony canal and be wide enough to support an anteriorly based flap that is directed through the new meatus and sutured to a cuff of periosteum at the glenoid fossa to serve as the anterolateral canal wall skin.

The conchal bowl and tragal complex aid in the proper placement of the new meatus and must be preserved by the otologist. If conchal cartilage is present during meatoplasty, the opening should be about 1.5 times the normal size because the cartilage helps resist meatal narrowing. However, if there is no conchal cartilage, the new meatus must be twice the normal size in anticipation of some postoperative stenosis.

The otologic and reconstructive surgeons must be aware that atresia surgery can adversely affect the appearance of the reconstructed auricle. There may be a loss of lateral projection caused by contracture in the postauricular sulcus after surgery. Postoperative soft tissue swelling may also cause a temporary loss of definition of the auricle, which normally diminishes and returns to its original appearance after a few weeks.

For the patient undergoing Medpor repair, the atresia surgery goes first, so the conchal bowl and tragus are not an issue as the Medpor auricle is built around the meatus.

The Facial Nerve

Surgeons must not be complacent regarding an abnormal course of the facial nerve in patients with microtia/atresia. Facial nerve injuries are debilitating to the patient and must be avoided at all costs. Thankfully, injury to this nerve is rare (<0.5% incidence).[16] Understanding the possible aberrant courses is essential to preventing accidental injury. The facial nerve often takes a more anterior approach at the level of the second genu and mastoid segment in patients with atresia **(Fig. 7)**.[30] Although not the legal standard, facial nerve monitoring is essential in complex otologic surgeries, such as atresia repair.[4,31] During the preoperative assessment, if an aberrant facial nerve is noted to travel through the area where the new canal will be created or blocks access to the oval window, atresiaplasty should not be attempted.

Although the facial nerve is at its greatest risk of injury during atresia surgery, there are times when a superficial nerve may be damaged from soft tissue dissection or even retraction of the auricle.[4] The aberrant anterior facial nerve may exit into the glenoid fossa and be vulnerable to injury in the preauricular area. Additionally, it may lack a vertical (mastoid) segment and may present as

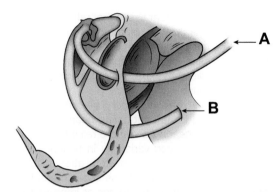

Fig. 7. Approximate course of intratemporal facial nerve in atretic ears. (*A*) Typical anterior course of the facial nerve in congenital aural atresia. (*B*) Normal course of the facial nerve. (*From* Crabtree JA. The facial nerve in congenital ear surgery. Otolaryngol Clin North Am 1974;7(2):505–10; with permission.)

soft tissue over the mastoid bone in patients with low-set ears. Surgery of the auricular framework may injure the nerve in this location. The nerve can also be stretched with overaggressive retraction of the auricle during atresia surgery or of the periauricular skin during microtia surgery. The frontal branch of the facial nerve can also be injured during the harvesting of a wide temporoparietal fascia flap in Medpor reconstruction.

Revision Surgery

An estimated 5% to 10% of patients undergoing canalplasty undergo a revision operation; common indications include loss of hearing, meatal stenosis, new bone growth, or loss of the skin graft with resultant mucosalization of the canal and a "wet" ear.[24] Revision canal surgery in the setting of rib graft microtia repair should not pose a problem because the cartilage graft recruits its own blood supply and heals if exposed. Conversely, the otologic surgeon must take care not to expose the Medpor framework during revision atresia surgery; the skin does not heal over this exposed area, and the child will need another procedure for coverage.

SUMMARY

Reconstruction of congenital microtia and aural atresia are some of the most challenging surgeries and require unique knowledge and experience. Evaluation of hearing status is essential in patients with CAA, and early auditory habilitation is important, especially in patients with bilateral microtia/atresia where a bone conducting hearing device is a necessity to support normal speech and language development. The role of bone conducting devices in patients with unilateral microtia/atresia is unclear.

When an osseointegrated bone conduction hearing device has been recommended or chosen by the family, it should be placed so as not to interfere with the surgical field of the reconstructive surgeon and so as not to cause feedback by touching or resting on the repaired auricle. The microtia repair is safest in this setting when performed before (or at the same time as) placement of the osseointegrated device.

Microtia surgery with rib grafting should precede atresiaplasty; however, atresiaplasty should precede microtia repair when Medpor is used. Surgeons must be aware of potential aberrant locations of the facial nerve to prevent injury. Revision canalplasty is undertaken safely with the rib graft reconstruction, but the otologist must be extremely careful not to expose the Medpor framework if the child has undergone Medpor microtia repair. It is imperative that the reconstructive surgeon and the otologist work together to achieve the best possible functional and cosmetic outcome.

REFERENCES

1. Jahrsdoerfer RA. Congenital atresia of the ear. Laryngoscope 1978;88(9 Pt 3 Suppl 13):1–48.
2. Service GJ, Roberson JB Jr. Current concepts in repair of aural atresia. Curr Opin Otolaryngol Head Neck Surg 2010;18(6):536–8.
3. Kesser B, Jahrsdoerfer R. Surgery for congenital aural atresia. In: Julianna Gulya A, Minor L, Poe D, editors. Surgery of the ear. 6th edition. Shelton (CT): People's Medical Publishing House; 2010. p. 413–22.
4. Jahrsdoerfer RA, Kesser BW. Issues on aural atresia for the facial plastic surgeon. Facial Plast Surg 1995; 11(4):274–7.
5. Kesser BW, Krook K, Gray LC. Impact of unilateral conductive hearing loss due to aural atresia on academic performance in children. Laryngoscope 2013;123(9):2270–5.
6. Yellon RF. Atresiaplasty versus BAHA for congenital aural atresia. Laryngoscope 2011;121(1):2–3.
7. Nadaraja GS, Gurgel RK, Kim J, et al. Hearing outcomes of atresia surgery versus osseointegrated bone conduction device in patients with congenital aural atresia: a systematic review. Otol Neurotol 2013;34(8):1394–9.
8. Evans AK, Kazahaya K. Canal atresia: "surgery or implantable hearing devices? the expert's question is revisited". Int J Pediatr Otorhinolaryngol 2007; 71(3):367–74.
9. Ricci G, Volpe AD, Faralli M, et al. Bone-anchored hearing aids (BAHA) in congenital aural atresia: personal experience. Int J Pediatr Otorhinolaryngol 2011;75(3):342–6.
10. Jahrsdoerfer RA, Yeakley JW, Aguilar EA, et al. Grading system for the selection of patients with congenital aural atresia. Am J Otol 1992;13:6–12.
11. Shonka DC Jr, Livingston WJ 3rd, Kesser BW. The Jahrsdoerfer grading scale in surgery to repair congenital aural atresia. Arch Otolaryngol Head Neck Surg 2008;134(8):873–7.
12. Oliver ER, Lambert PR, Rumboldt Z, et al. Middle ear dimensions in congenital aural atresia and hearing outcomes after atresiaplasty. Otol Neurotol 2010; 31(6):946–53.
13. Nicholas BD, Krook KA, Gray LC, et al. Does preoperative hearing predict postoperative hearing in patients undergoing primary aural atresia repair? Otol Neurotol 2012;33(6):1002–6.
14. Lambert PR. Congenital aural atresia: stability of surgical results. Laryngoscope 1998;108(12):1801–5.
15. De la Cruz A, Teufert KB. Congenital aural atresia surgery: long-term results. Otolaryngol Head Neck Surg 2003;129(1):121–7.
16. Li CL, Dai PD, Yang L, et al. A meta-analysis of the long-term hearing outcomes and complications associated with atresiaplasty. Int J Pediatr Otorhinolaryngol 2015;79(6):793–7.
17. Brent B. Auricular repair with autogenous rib cartilage grafts: two decades of experience with 600 cases. Plast Reconstr Surg 1992;90(3):355–74 [discussion: 375–6].
18. Brent B. Technical advances in ear reconstruction with autogenous rib cartilage grafts: personal experience with 1200 cases. Plast Reconstr Surg 1999; 104(2):319–34 [discussion: 335–8].
19. Nagata S. Modification of the stages in total reconstruction of the auricle. Part I. grafting the three-dimensional costal cartilage framework for lobule-type microtia. Plast Reconstr Surg 1994;93(2):221–30 [discussion: 267–8].
20. Cho BC, Kim JY, Byun JS. Two-stage reconstruction of the auricle in congenital microtia using autogenous costal cartilage. J Plast Reconstr Aesthet Surg 2007;60(9):998–1006.
21. Yellon RF. Combined atresiaplasty and tragal reconstruction for microtia and congenital aural atresia: thesis for the American Laryngological, Rhinological, and Otological Society. Laryngoscope 2009; 119(2):245–54.
22. Roberson JB Jr, Reinisch J, Colen TY, et al. Atresia repair before microtia reconstruction: comparison of early with standard surgical timing. Otol Neurotol 2009;30(6):771–6.
23. Ahn J, Baek SY, Kim K, et al. Predictive factors for hearing outcomes after canalplasty in patients with congenital aural atresia. Otol Neurotol 2017; 38(8):1140–4.
24. Oliver ER, Hughley BB, Shonka DC, et al. Revision aural atresia surgery: indications and outcomes. Otol Neurotol 2011;32(2):252–8.

25. Kesser BW, Cole ED, Gray LC. Emergence of binaural summation after surgical correction of unilateral congenital aural atresia. Otol Neurotol 2016; 37(5):499–503.

26. Gray L, Kesser B, Cole E. Understanding speech in noise after correction of congenital unilateral aural atresia: effects of age in the emergence of binaural squelch but not in use of head-shadow. Int J Pediatr Otorhinolaryngol 2009;73(9):1281–7.

27. Byun H, Moon IJ, Woo SY, et al. Objective and subjective improvement of hearing in noise after surgical correction of unilateral congenital aural atresia in pediatric patients: a prospective study using the hearing in noise test, the sound-spatial-quality questionnaire, and the Glasgow benefit inventory. Ear Hear 2015;36(4):e183–9.

28. Moon IJ, Byun H, Jin SH, et al. Sound localization performance improves after canaloplasty in unilateral congenital aural atresia patients. Otol Neurotol 2014;35(4):639–44.

29. Casale G, Nicholas BD, Kesser BW. Acquired ear canal cholesteatoma in congenital aural atresia/stenosis. Otol Neurotol 2014;35(8):1474–9.

30. Crabtree JA. The facial nerve in congenital ear surgery. Otolaryngol Clin North Am 1974;7(2):505–10.

31. Ruhl DS, Hong SS, Littlefield PD. Lessons learned in otologic surgery: 30 years of malpractice cases in the United States. Otol Neurotol 2013;34(7):1173–9.

Auricular Prostheses in Microtia

Philippe A. Federspil, MD

KEYWORDS

• Bone anchorage • Osseointegration • Titanium implant • Silicone • Ear prosthesis • Pinna

KEY POINTS

- Modern silicones as well as osseointegrated titanium implants allow for rehabilitation of patients with microtia with an inconspicuous auricular prosthesis.
- Computer science with virtual planning and rapid prototyping is about to revolutionize the process of prosthetic auricular rehabilitation.
- The state of the art for prosthetic rehabilitation is the use of osseointegrated percutaneous implants.
- Auricular prostheses may be used as a temporary measure, a rescue procedure in failed auricular (re)construction, or as a definitive treatment option.
- Auricular prostheses are not just an alternative but also a viable treatment option for patients with microtia.

INTRODUCTION

An auricular prosthesis is an artificial substitute for malformed, lost, or removed parts of the pinna. In the German and Scandinavian linguistic area, the word *episthesis* is preferred in order to stress that these types of prostheses are placed on top of facial skin. The art of making craniofacial prostheses is called anaplastology. Virtually all available materials, for example, porcelain, wax, rubber, and paper mache, have been used in the long history of anaplastology.[1] Obviously, the major drawbacks for rehabilitation with auricular prostheses were the use of inadequate material and the lack of reliable methods for retention. The breakthrough for ear prostheses came with the introduction of the modern silicones and its colorings. The movie industry had a tremendous impact on the evolution of silicones used for body masks. Silicone is flexible and keeps the body temperature. Hair and pigments can be introduced into the material. Its edges can be made so thin as to become transparent, in such a way that the prosthesis blends into the face, which enhances the camouflage even more. Moreover, the prosthesis can be made as a mirrored replica of the opposite side and be adapted to patients' wishes. Digital color scanning of the skin complexion aids the anaplastologist in matching the skin to the coloring of the prosthesis. Computer science has reached the planning, modeling, and manufacturing of craniofacial prostheses.[2] Laser surface scanning, image processing of computed tomography (CT) data with virtual mirroring, and rapid prototyping with 3-dimensional printing are some of the currently used tools. Exact templates for correct implant position can be made. Molds can be printed out based on mirrored images of the healthy contralateral auricle. Therefore, not only the position of the implants and prosthesis can be optimized but also the whole process is likely to be revolutionized in the near future.

The author has received travel grants from Cochlear Ltd. as well as Medicon eG, and is involved in implant development for Medicon eG.
Department of Oto-Rhino-Laryngology, University Hospital Heidelberg, INF 400, Heidelberg 69120, Germany
E-mail address: federspil@med.uni-heidelberg.de

Facial Plast Surg Clin N Am 26 (2018) 97–104
https://doi.org/10.1016/j.fsc.2017.09.007
1064-7406/18/© 2017 Elsevier Inc. All rights reserved.

COUNSELING OF PATIENTS WITH MICROTIA

In general, the management of patients with existing or impending auricular defects depends to a large extent on (1) the cause of the auricular deficit with its associated factors (eg, radiotherapy in patients with cancer), (2) the age of patients, (3) the medical comorbidities, (4) the patients' ethnic and cultural background, as well as (5) psychological issues.[3] The prosthetic options should be discussed with patients (and parents) in a team approach with the anaplastologist, including the need for osseointegrated implants to ensure retention. Additional malformations, as in the Treacher-Collins syndrome, have to be included in the treatment plan.

Probably the most important factor in counseling is patients' age, thereby their ability for their own informed consent. Often, children develop a sense of malformation only at the 10 years of age. However, some patients with microtia without the associated malformation cope very well and do not wish to have anything done. However, puberty may change views. Definitively, counseling of these patients and their parents requires time and dedication to elaborate all of the aforementioned aspects of care. Sometimes children can be managed quite well with an adhesive-retained auricular prosthesis. This prosthesis may serve as an interim solution before any of the available options, but it also helps the child/adolescent in the process of decision-making (**Figs. 1** and **2**).

Implant surgery creates scars that preclude plastic reconstructive surgery with rib cartilage. Although the temporoparietal fascia flap may still be available if the superficial temporal vessels were spared, undoubtedly reconstructive surgery is much more difficult if at all possible. Therefore, the author prefers to postpone implant surgery until adolescents are mature enough to judge the consequences and risks of either surgery and are able to make the decision themselves.

On the other hand, rehabilitation with implant-retained ear prosthesis always remains an option even in the case of failed reconstruction. In the author's experience, it is best if the candidate meets a patient with an ear prosthesis in the clinic. Often, this eliminates fears of skin-penetrating implants and the artificial nature of the prosthesis. However, it also clarifies the need for implant hygiene and all aspects of life with an auricular prosthesis. Although the prosthesis has to be considered to be a foreign body, astonishingly, patients accept it as part of their body. The greatest advantage of the ear prosthesis is that it can be manufactured as a mirrored replica of the opposite side.

It is important to note that not every child with microtia needs a temporary auricular prosthesis. There are many patients who are psychologically stable and do not want any form of treatment. Careful evaluation of young patients' wishes and views is mandatory, as they may differ from those of the parents.

The medical comorbidities have to be taken into consideration: An absolute contraindication for implant surgery is severe psychiatric disease (eg, severe dementia) and bad medical condition. Poor hygiene, drug/alcohol addiction, and mild psychiatric disease are relative contraindications.

The advantages of auricular prostheses in patients with microtia are[3]

- Simple and fast method
- Optimal camouflage
- Predictable cosmetic result (can be shown before surgery)
- Extremely thin prosthetic edges to become transparent and blend into the face, thereby augmenting camouflage (less wear off when implants are used)
- No donor site morbidity
- Secure retention provided by osseointegrated implants

The disadvantages of auricular prostheses are[3]

- Prostheses are not ideal for the replacement of mobile parts of the face; in the auricular region, this plays a lesser role; however, jaw movements with the mouth opening have to be considered.

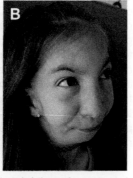

Fig. 1. (*A*) A 9-year-old girl with bilateral anotia and sequelae of complicated mandibular distraction. (*B*) Adhesive-retained auricular prosthesis made of silicone (anaplastologist Mathias Schneider, Zweibrücken, Germany). (*From* Federspil PA. The role of auricular prostheses (epitheses) in ear reconstruction. Facial Plast Surg 2015;31(6):627; with permission.)

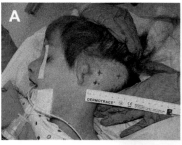
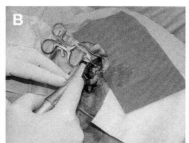
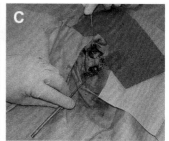
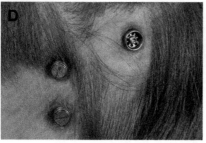
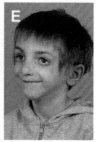

Fig. 2. (*A*) A 7-year-old boy with Treacher-Collins syndrome. Planned implant positions for bone-anchored prosthesis and hearing aid. The mother is also wearing implant-retained auricular prostheses. (*B*) Insertion of a Vistafix 3 implant by Cochlear Ltd. (*C*) Two implants for the prosthesis and one for the hearing aid in place. (*D*) Implant site after healing. Two Technovent O-ring magnets in place. (*E*) Boy with fitted (bilateral) auricular prosthesis (anaplastologist Norbert Schilling, Neubrunn, Germany).

- The prosthesis is a foreign body and has to be taken off at night.
- There might be a color mismatch with changing complexion and UV exposure or discoloring by cigarette smoke.
- There is a lifelong renewal of the prosthesis required, usually every 2 to 3 years, adding to its cost.
- When implants are used, the skin penetration site needs regular cleaning.

AURICULAR PROSTHESES AS A TEMPORARY MEASURE

Auricular prostheses can be used in children and adolescents with microtia as a temporary measure while waiting for reconstructive surgery or for testing before implant surgery.[4] In both situations, the prosthesis is fixed by the use of medical adhesives on top of the auricular remnant. Usually, the fabrication of the cosmetically appealing prosthesis is more feasible the smaller the remnant. In large remnants, it may be difficult to integrate the remnant underneath the prosthesis and still provide an inconspicuous prosthesis in an anatomically correct position. Possible drawbacks include adverse effects by the medical adhesive, improper position depending on the remnant, less reliable fixation, and difficult positioning. Generally speaking, the remnant should be removed in order to obtain an optimal cosmetic result with the auricular prosthesis. However, this is of course not warranted in patients awaiting reconstructive surgery. Still, far ectopic auricular remnants sometimes have to be surgically removed because they cannot be integrated into the prosthesis.

Auricular prostheses can also be used for testing before implant surgery. Usually, this is not necessary in adults. However, in children and adolescents, it is advisable, especially in the process of deciding whether reconstructive surgery or implant surgery should be chosen. The period of the temporary measure might extend for years in this situation.

AURICULAR PROSTHESES AS A RESCUE PROCEDURE IN FAILED RECONSTRUCTION

As a rule, prosthetic treatment can always be offered to patients. Therefore, patients with failed reconstruction may be rescued by the use of auricular prostheses. Although this indication was quite common a few decades ago, it has become much less frequent with the evolution of surgical techniques in auricular reconstruction. However, it still occurs to some degree because patients' estimation and the objective view of the result may differ in either way. If patients have come to the conclusion that they opt to convert to prosthetic rehabilitation, usually the constructed framework has to be removed, while local skin is sufficient for closure after implant placement (**Fig. 3**).

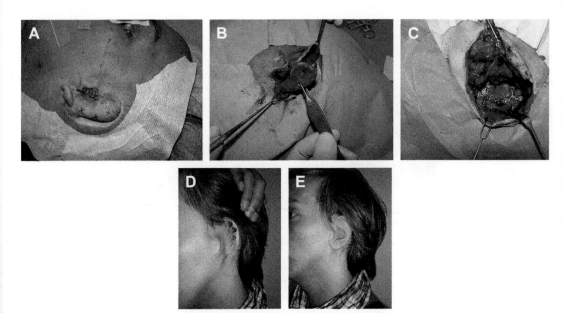

Fig. 3. (*A*) A 25-year-old patient after failed ear reconstruction in grade III unilateral microtia. Surgical planning of implant positions. (*B*) The cartilage framework had to be removed. (*C*) Placement of an ear plate of the Epi-plating system by Medicon e.G. (Tuttlingen, Germany) with 3 abutment threads. (*D*) Implant site with 3 magnets for coupling. (*E*) The patient with an implant-retained auricular prosthesis (anaplastologist Jörn Brom, Heidelberg, Germany). (*From* Federspil PA. The role of auricular prostheses (epitheses) in ear reconstruction. Facial Plast Surg 2015;31(6):626–32; with permission.)

AURICULAR PROSTHESES AS A DEFINITIVE TREATMENT OPTION

It is the patients' right to choose prosthetic rehabilitation as a definitive treatment.[5] There are many patients with microtia who chose implant-retained auricular prosthesis without any previous reconstructive surgery. Adults can give their informed consent after careful counseling. Models of auricular serve to show the anaplastologist's skill and artwork. They can go for adhesive-retained prostheses without any surgical risk, if they are willing to take the inconvenience and unpredictability of medical adhesives. However, there is a clear benefit of using osseointegrated implants for retention, making this the treatment of choice. As mentioned earlier, this process is more difficult in children and adolescents. Children with microtia can and have been successfully rehabilitated with implant-retained ear prostheses in various institutions, including the author's own.[6,7] However, the question remains if this is appropriate in the light of the advances in reconstructive surgery. Usually, the combination with bone-anchored hearing aids (BAHA by Cochlear, Ltd, Mölnlycke, Sweden or Ponto by Oticon Medical, Inc, Askim, Sweden) poses no difficulties nor does it preclude reconstructive surgery.[8] However, difficulties in placing implants for

prostheses may arise, when other implantable hearing devices have been previously used, which involve removing bone in the mastoid region. Therefore, the surgeon should consider the future option for an implant-retained auricular prosthesis when counseling patients and parents about hearing restoration.

OPTIONS FOR RETENTION OF AURICULAR PROSTHESES

Generally, craniofacial prostheses can be retained in different ways:

1. *Anatomic anchorage*: The prosthesis is retained by undercuts of the defect in which it is squeezed in like a mushroom. This method may work in the orbit, but the ear canal if present never allows reliable fixation.
2. *Mechanical anchorage*: Various mechanical devices, such as head springs, have been tried with little success. Spectacle frames do not provide enough strength to keep auricular prostheses in place unless aided otherwise.
3. *Chemical anchorage*: Medical-grade adhesives may provide satisfactory fixation for a limited time period of a couple of hours. Retention degrades over time by perspiration, transpiration, and other environmental factors. Furthermore,

dermal irritation from long-term contact with occlusion or allergic reaction is not uncommon with the use of adhesives. The main companies selling adhesives for silicone prostheses are Factor II, Inc (Lakeside, AZ) and Technovent Ltd (Bridgend, UK). Another drawback of adhesive-retained prostheses is that they deteriorate more quickly and have to be renewed usually every year.

4. *Surgical anchorage:* Bone-anchorage by osseointegrated implants provided a major breakthrough for prostheses because this method guarantees secure and reliable retention.[9] As compared with adhesives, the main advantages of bone anchorage are

   a. The retention is not influenced by environmental factors.

   b. The auricular prostheses is easily mounted in the correct position by patients themselves because of the use of magnets or the bar construction.

   c. The convenience of wearing is improved by not using adhesives and less skin occlusion.

   d. The functional life for implant-retained auricular prostheses is extended, because the wear off on the edges due to the daily application and removal of adhesives is eliminated.

OSSEOINTEGRATION

In the 1950s, Per-Ingvar Brånemark and colleagues[10] made the discovery of the tremendous biocompatibility of titanium in bone and coined the expression "osseointegration."[10] At first, osseointegration was defined as direct contact to bone as examined by light microscopy. However, it was found that the bone contact area in osseointegrated implants was only 70% to 80% on average.[11] On electron microscopy, there is an amorphous gap of 20 to 500 nm. The clinical definition given by Zarb und Albrektsson[12] still holds true today: "*A process whereby clinically asymptomatic rigid fixation of alloplastic materials is achieved, and maintained, in bone during functional loading.*" Factors that influence the establishment of osseointegration include (1) biocompatibility, (2) implant design, (3) implant surface, (4) condition of recipient area, (5) surgical technique, and (6) implant loading.[13]

The first time titanium implants were used percutaneously outside the oral cavity was 1977 by Anders Tjellström and colleagues[14] for a bone-anchored hearing aid. Two years later, in 1979, the first bone-anchored ear prosthesis was provided for a patient.[15] Bone anchorage has significant advantages over the other methods of retention.[16]

IMPLANT SYSTEMS

The extraoral implant systems are derived from dental implants. The first system was the Brånemark system, which is a solitary screw-type implant made out of commercially pure titanium (cp Ti) with a minimally rough surface. The American Society for Testing and Materials (ASTM) provides the specification F-67 for unalloyed titanium as a surgical implant with the grades 1 to 4. Although most osteosynthesis plates are produced according to ASTM F-67, various titanium alloys, such as the very popular alloy titanium-6aluminium-4vanadium (Ti6Al4V), are used in orthopedic titanium implants that have to bear more strain. Ti6Al4V bone screws have been shown a comparable bone contact area to unalloyed titanium implants in animal experiments[17] and retrieved human specimens.[18]

Although there is great diversity of implant systems and manufacturers for dental implants, there are only few systems available for prostheses. In order to group the available systems, the terms *solitary* and *grouped* implants have been introduced. Among other systems derived from the original Brånemark implant, for example, Straumann (Oticon Medical Inc, Askim, Sweden) or Southern Implants (Irene, Centurion, RSA), the most widely used solitary implant is currently marketed under the name Vistafix by Cochlear, Ltd. It consists of self-tapping screws (flange fixture) with a moderately rough surface for faster osseointegration. They are 4 mm in diameter and come in 2 lengths: 3 mm or 4 mm. There is a new magnet attachment with an O-Ring by Technovent, Ltd (Bridgend, UK) that combines magnetic and mechanical retention.

Grouped implant systems consist of a platelike titanium implant, which is placed underneath the periosteum. These implants are fixed to the bone with several titanium bone screws according to the technique of osteosynthesis. Thereby, the loading forces are spread to multiple, or grouped, bone screws. This allows implantation in areas with anatomically unfavorable bony resources, for example, the well pneumatized mastoid. The only system that is currently available is the Epiplating system. It was developed in 2000 by the Medicon eG company (Tuttlingen, Germany) in collaboration with P. Federspil, Ph.A. Federspil, und M. Schneider.[19] The system is approved for usage in Europe (CE mark). However, the company did not apply for its approval by the FDA in the United States. It is the adaptation of the 2.0 titanium miniplate system used in craniofacial trauma care to the needs of anaplastology. The plates are made of grade 2 unalloyed titanium according to ASTM F-67, that is, cp Ti. The bone screws are made of Ti6Al4V according to ASTM F-136. The system comes with specialized plates for different anatomic regions. They are 1 mm in height but 2 mm in width, therefore, somewhat more resistant to strain by loading and less vulnerable by mobility. The tapped holes for percutaneous abutments are 2 mm in height, therefore, providing good retention of the elements screwed in.

A common feature of all currently available systems is that they require a percutaneous connection. The connecting part through the skin is called abutment or base post. The auricular prosthesis may be connected to the implants either by the classic clip-bar system or by magnets. The bar construction requires parallel implant axes to a large extent. Otherwise it is virtually impossible to produce a bar that does not put strain on the implants.[20] However, retentive clips may be adjusted in strength to individual needs. On the other hand, magnets are easier to clean.[21] An inconvenience is that magnets have to be removed before using MRI.

PLANNING IMPLANT POSITION

The area of placement has to be chosen according to the needs of the anaplastologist regardless of the implant system in use. It is wise to discuss the case in a team approach. Usually, 2 percutaneous abutments provide sufficient retention for a bar construction. However, for magnets, more often 3 is chosen. The ideal position of the percutaneous connection is approximately 20 mm from the center of the outer ear canal, or in an atretic ear, the anticipated opening. Classically, the positions are at 8:00 and 10:30 on the right side, when projecting a clock on patients. On the left side, this corresponds to 4:00 and 1:30. However, in the author's, experience it is preferable to place the lower implant at 9:00 or, 3:00, respectively. In all cases, the minimum distance between abutments or magnets should be 15 mm. The area of percutaneous abutments reflects the location of the antihelix.

SURGICAL TECHNIQUE

The basic principles of implant surgery were all elaborated in the original Brånemark technique. The surgery consists of 2 steps: step 1 is the placement of the implant, and step 2 is the soft tissue reduction and percutaneous connection. Originally, the two procedures were separated by a healing period of 3 months with the implant unloaded. Steps 1 and 2 may be combined to a single-stage procedure in adult patients with a cortical bone width of more than 3 mm and no history of radiotherapy. Then the healing period may

be reduced to 6 weeks. However, in children, it still is kept longer at even 6 months. Minimizing trauma to the bone is of paramount importance by (1) the use of a sharp burr, (2) low drilling speed at 1500 to 2000 rpm, and (3) ample cooling with saline solution.

For solitary implants, palpating movements while drilling with a Rosen burr allows for controlling the bone width and detection of the dura. In a well-pneumatized mastoid, it often happens to enter mastoid air sells. It might even be difficult to find enough bone width at the desired implantation site. The burr hole is then widened by a spiral drill. The self-tapping titanium fixture is inserted with the machine at low speed under torque control (10–45 Ncm). The titanium fixture should only be handled with titanium instruments in order to avoid contamination. The longer fixture is preferred. At this point, the inner threads of the implant are now secured by a cover screw, and the wound is closed, if the procedure is conducted in 2 steps. Radical soft tissue reduction was considered essential in order to avoid adverse skin reactions at the implant site. However, this attitude is about to change, as it did in implant surgery for bone conduction hearing systems. The skin is removed by a biopsy punch over the implant, and the skin penetrating the abutment is inserted under torque control with 25 Ncm. An abutment clamp provides counter torque in order not to move the underlying implant. Ointment soaked ribbon gauze is wrapped around the abutment under a healing cap in order to avoid the formation of a hematoma.

For grouped implant systems, standard osteosynthesis instruments are used with the addition of a few special tools. The bony surface is exposed while preserving a periosteal flap. In the Epiplating system, several implant options are available: (1) ear plate with 2 threaded holes, (2) ear plate with 3 threaded holes, or (3) universal plates. The plate is bent to meet the bony contour. Moreover, it may be cut to meet special anatomic situations. Before doing so, the threads are secured by cover screws in order to avoid any distortion that would impact on mounting the abutments into the threaded holes. The plate is held at the desired position, and a hole for the bone screw is created by a 1.6-mm spiral drill at low speed under ample cooling. Care is taken while inserting the self-tapping bone screw in order to minimize trauma and strain on the bone. A minimum of 3 bone screws is used per plate. Soft tissue reduction is performed very conservatively if at all, aiming at preserving a maximum of viable tissue. Percutaneous abutments (so-called base posts) are inserted. Magnets may be mounted onto the abutments or

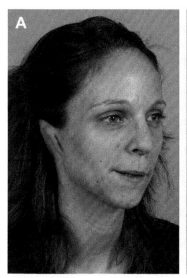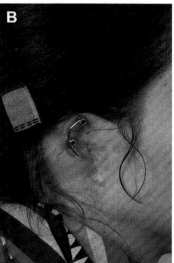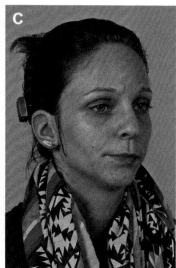

Fig. 4. (*A*) A 29-year-old patient with grade III unilateral microtia. No previous treatment. (*B*) Close-up view of the implant site with a bar construction on 2 percutaneous abutments mounted on Epiplating CMS implants. (*C*) The patient with an implant-retained auricular prosthesis (anaplastologist Mathias Schneider, Zweibrücken, Germany). The patient has simultaneously been fitted with a BAHA on a BI300 implant without soft tissue reduction. (*From* Federspil PA. The role of auricular prostheses (epitheses) in ear reconstruction. Facial Plast Surg 2015;31(6):631; with permission.)

inserted directly into the plate. Unlike the solitary implants, the plate systems are resistant to torque with abutment insertion (**Fig. 4**).

OUTCOME FOR IMPLANT-RETAINED AURICULAR PROSTHESES

The largest experience worldwide has been gathered with the Brånemark system. The highest rates of osseointegration with extraoral implantation are obtained in the mastoid in comparison with other sites in the facial skeleton. The success rates with regard to implant survival range from 95%[22] to 99%[23] in the nonirradiated temporal bone. Parel and Tjellström[24] report a success rate of 98.3%. Wolfaardt and colleagues[25] had a 98.9% success rate in the same region. In the author's own institution, the success rate is 97.7% for Brånemark implants for auricular prostheses[26] and 100% for 27 Epiplating implants.

The adverse skin reactions can be graded according to the Holgers score[27] whereby 0 is no reaction, 1 is reddish, 2 is red and moist, 3 is granulation tissue, and 4 is skin infection to such a degree that the abutment has to be removed. A Swedish study reported 92.5% of patients with a bone-anchored hearing implant had a Holgers score of 0 and 89.3% of patients with auricular prostheses, respectively.[27] There is rarely any discomfort around the implant. Cleaning with mild soap is crucial. If a skin irritation occurs, the abutment should be checked for loosening, as this might open a space to harbor bacterial biofilm.

SUMMARY

The progress made in the development of the silicones as well as percutaneous titanium implants allow for rehabilitation of patients with microtia with an inconspicuous auricular prosthesis (or ear episthesis). The art of making the prosthesis by the dedicated anaplastologist is the key for the success of this approach. Most patients with microtia desire camouflage. The greatest advantage of the auricular prosthesis is that it can be manufactured as a mirrored replica of the opposite side. Computer science with virtual planning and rapid prototyping is about to revolutionize the process of prosthetic auricular rehabilitation.

Auricular prostheses may be used as a temporary measure, a rescue procedure in failed auricular (re)construction, or as a definitive treatment option. Conventional retention by medical-grade adhesives, sometimes helped by making use of the remnant, keeps its place in the use as a temporary measure or if patients decline surgery. However, the state of the art for prosthetic rehabilitation is the use of osseointegrated percutaneous implants because they provide the best retention as well as easy mounting by the patients themselves and longer preservation of the fine transparent edges of the prostheses that augment camouflage. Over all, auricular prostheses are not just an alternative but also a viable treatment option for patients with microtia.

REFERENCES

1. Ring ME. The history of maxillofacial prosthetics. Plast Reconstr Surg 1991;87(1):174–84.
2. Ariani N, Visser A, van Oort RP, et al. Current state of craniofacial prosthetic rehabilitation. Int J Prosthodont 2013;26(1):57–67.
3. Federspil PA. Implant-retained craniofacial prostheses for facial defects. GMS Curr Top Otorhinolaryngol Head Neck Surg 2009;8:Doc03.
4. Federspil PA. The role of auricular prostheses (epitheses) in ear reconstruction. Facial Plast Surg 2015;31(6):626–32.
5. Federspil PA. Ear epitheses as an alternative to autogenous reconstruction. Facial Plast Surg 2009; 25(3):190–203.
6. Han K, Son D. Osseointegrated alloplastic ear reconstruction with the implant-carrying plate system in children. Plast Reconstr Surg 2002;109(2): 496–503 [discussion: 504–5].
7. Granstrom G, Bergstrom K, Odersjo M, et al. Osseointegrated implants in children: experience from our first 100 patients. Otolaryngol Head Neck Surg 2001;125(1):85–92.
8. Federspil PA, Koch A, Schneider MH, et al. Percutaneous titanium implants for bone conduction hearing aids: experience with 283 cases. HNO 2014;62(7): 490–7 [in German].
9. Federspil P, Federspil PA. Prosthetic management of craniofacial defects. HNO 1998;46(6):569–78 [in German].
10. Brånemark PI, Hansson BO, Adell R, et al. Osseointegrated implants in the treatment of edentulous jaw. Experience from a 10-year period. Scand J Plast Reconstr Surg 1977;11(Suppl 16):1–175.
11. Albrektsson T, Eriksson AR, Friberg B, et al. Histologic investigations on 33 retrieved Nobelpharma implants. Clin Mater 1993;12(1):1–9.
12. Zarb GA, Albrektsson T. Osseointegration - a requiem for the periodontal ligament? Int J Periodontics Restorative Dent 1991;11(1):88–91.
13. Albrektsson T, Brånemark PI, Hansson HA, et al. Osseointegrated titanium implants. Requirements for ensuring a long-lasting, direct bone-to-implant anchorage in man. Acta Orthop Scand 1981;52(2): 155–70.
14. Tjellström A, Lindström J, Hallen O, et al. Osseointegrated titanium implants in the temporal bone. A clinical study on bone-anchored hearing aids. Am J Otol 1981;2(4):304–10.
15. Tjellström A, Lindström J, Nylen O, et al. The bone-anchored auricular episthesis. Laryngoscope 1981; 91(5):811–5.
16. Toljanic JA, Eckert SE, Roumanas E, et al. Osseointegrated craniofacial implants in the rehabilitation of orbital defects: an update of a retrospective experience in the United States. J Prosthet Dent 2005; 94(2):177–82.
17. Schön R, Schmelzeisen R, Shirota T, et al. Tissue reaction around miniplates used for the fixation of vascularized iliac crest bone grafts. Oral Surg Oral Med Oral Pathol Oral Radiol Endod 1997;83(4):433–40.
18. Hwang K, Schmitt JM, Hollinger JO. Interface between titanium miniplate/screw and human calvaria. J Craniofac Surg 2000;11(2):184–8.
19. Federspil PA, Plinkert PK. Knochenverankerte Hörgeräte immer beidseitig! HNO 2002;50(5):405–9.
20. Miller KL, Faulkner G, Wolfaardt JF. Misfit and functional loading of craniofacial implants. Int J Prosthodont 2004;17(3):267–73.
21. Federspil PA, Federspil P, Schneider MH. Magnetverankerung in der Epithetik. In: Blankenstein F, editor. Magnete in der Zahnmedizin. Rottweil (Germany): Flohr verlag; 2001. p. 104–9.
22. Watson RM, Coward TJ, Forman GH. Results of treatment of 20 patients with implant-retained auricular prostheses. Int J Oral Maxillofac Implants 1995; 10(4):445–9.
23. Tolman DE, Taylor PF. Bone-anchored craniofacial prosthesis study: irradiated patients. Int J Oral Maxillofac Implants 1996;11(5):612–9.
24. Parel SM, Tjellström A. The United States and Swedish experience with osseointegration and facial prostheses. Int J Oral Maxillofac Implants 1991; 6(1):75–9.
25. Wolfaardt JF, Wilkes GH, Parel SM, et al. Craniofacial osseointegration: the Canadian experience. Int J Oral Maxillofac Implants 1993;8(2):197–204.
26. Junker OH. Epithetische rehabilitation kraniofazialer Defekte. Eine Langzeituntersuchung über 12 Jahre bei 200 Patienten. Homburg (Germany): Universitäts-HNO-Klinik, Universität des Saarlandes; 2006.
27. Holgers KM, Roupe G, Tjellström A, et al. Clinical, immunological and bacteriological evaluation of adverse reactions to skin-penetrating titanium implants in the head and neck region. Contact Dermatitis 1992;27(1):1–7.

Moving?

Make sure your subscription moves with you!

To notify us of your new address, find your **Clinics Account Number** (located on your mailing label above your name), and contact customer service at:

Email: journalscustomerservice-usa@elsevier.com

800-654-2452 (subscribers in the U.S. & Canada)
314-447-8871 (subscribers outside of the U.S. & Canada)

Fax number: 314-447-8029

Elsevier Health Sciences Division
Subscription Customer Service
3251 Riverport Lane
Maryland Heights, MO 63043

ELSEVIER

Moving?

Make sure your subscription moves with you!

To notify us of your new address, find your Clinics Account Number (located on your mailing label above your name), and contact customer service at:

Email: journalscustomerservice-usa@elsevier.com

800-654-2452 (subscribers in the U.S. & Canada)
314-447-8871 (subscribers outside of the U.S. & Canada)

Fax number: 314-447-8029

Elsevier Health Sciences Division
Subscription Customer Service
3251 Riverport Lane
Maryland Heights, MO 63043

To ensure uninterrupted delivery of your subscription, please notify us at least 4 weeks in advance of move.